First Printing, 2023

DR HAISONG WANG AND
PRYOR HOLLIS

I KNOW YOU KNOW

INTEGRATING TRADITIONAL AND CONTEMPORARY HEALING THINKING AND APPLICATION

The Healthy Influence Books

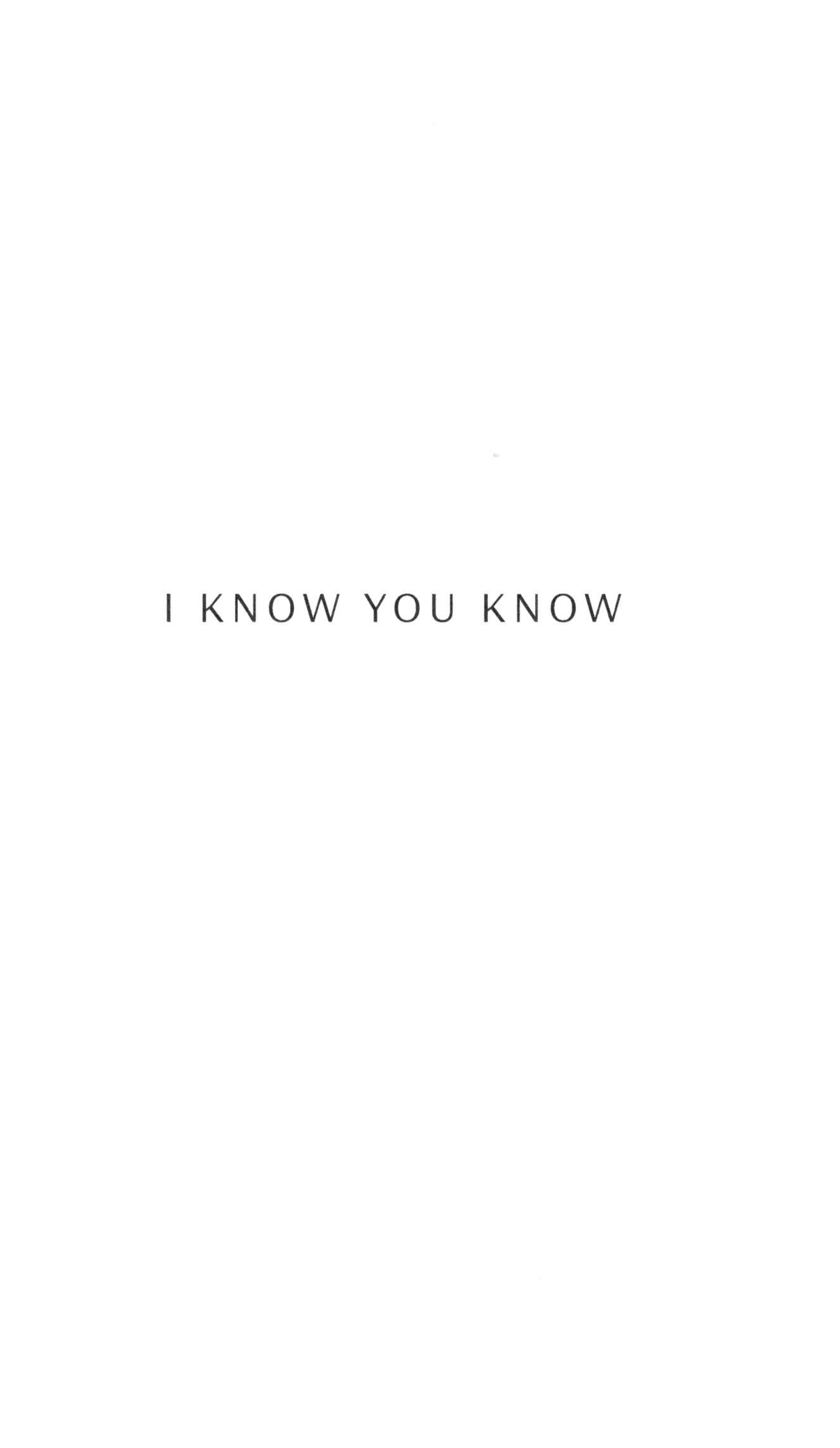

I KNOW YOU KNOW

To our ever-expansive, yet interconnected health community.

Our understanding of health and wellbeing stems from your willingness to share your unique perspectives and embrace new knowledge with an open mind. It is your motivation to heal and grow that inspires this book, and your trust in us and in yourselves is deeply humbling.

Thank you for taking this journey with us.

CONTENTS

CONTENTS

CONTENTS

INTRODUCING DR HAISONG WANG

My Chinese medicine journey dates back through generations of my family and heritage. My wife is also a Chinese medicine practitioner, as well as my father-in-law, mother, brother, and sister-in-law. We often work together, always learning from each other, and building on our shared generational knowledge. My journey is a collective journey.

The philosophies of Chinese medicine were surrounding me, from the very beginning, and formed a foundation of appreciation for and curiosity of Chinese medicine. Though it seemed natural for me to be drawn into the path of Chinese medicine, it was also my own passion that guided me towards this journey. I love to learn. For me, learning is not just necessary to put new knowledge into practice. It is an avenue of connection and appreciation for the world around us. My curiosity and interest in various topics inspire me to seek out answers, and in turn, the answers I find yield further questions. Learning is a journey, an attitude, and a way through which I can connect with the world.

Beyond this, I am also fascinated by different levels and ways of thinking and perceiving. Chinese medicine involves a wide- ranging level of thought, connecting ancient healing techniques and ideology with modern-day contexts. Today more than ever, the integration of Chinese medicine and mainstream modern medicine introduces yet another level of thought within this already expansive layer of healing.

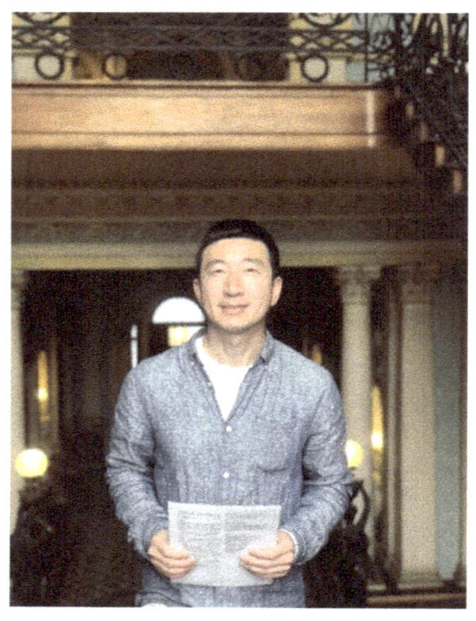

I started my career in medicine, working in an emergency department in China. Making life-or-death decisions and collaborating with others was a major part of my daily routine. I learned to assess the facts of situations and select the best path of care for patients within short amounts of time, knowing that there could be immediate life-changing consequences. This experience taught me to think and act logically, and embedded within me a new level of understanding of the value of human life, and how swiftly our health can take an unexpected turn. Though my work primarily took place during the most critical times of a patient's life, there were still moments in which I would care for patients before and after their treatment in the emergency department. I started to see a more holistic way of caring and healing, that stretched across lives far beyond the most urgent moments.

Upon moving to Canberra, Australia, around twenty five years ago, I faced a new language, a new environment, and a new job. Additionally, having to work independently as a Chinese medicine practitioner meant I had more limited resources than I had in China – I had to be resilient and adaptive.

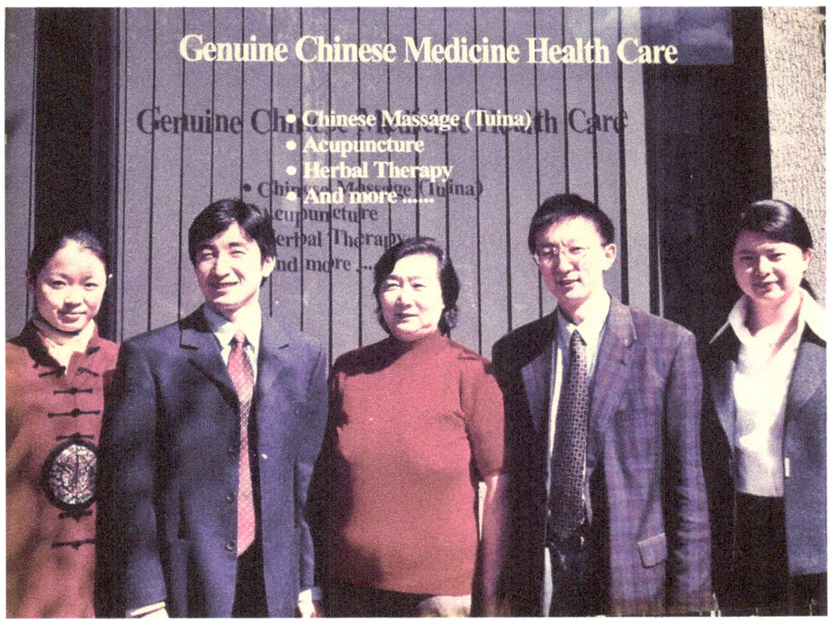

At the time, the Canberra Institute of Technology (CIT) was looking to expand their teaching opportunities in Chinese medicine and connected with the hospital where I was working. I was given the opportunity to start as a teacher for Technical and Further Education (TAFE) courses in Chinese medicine at the CIT. Not only was the course fast-paced and highly practical, but it also required me to teach in English for the first time. I quickly developed strategies to simultaneously learn and apply the English language. As part of the course, I also regularly took CIT students back to China to practice their skills in Chinese medicine. The ten years I spent teaching flew by.

In the year 2000, my brother and I also opened our own practising clinic with the support of our family. We shared the same vision of progressing the Chinese medicine and holistic healthcare community in Australia. Through networking in the local community, we also collaborated with a group of health professionals with similar goals and values, including physiotherapists, psychologists, dentists, massage therapists, and other Chinese medicine experts and enthusiasts. To this day, we continue to learn from each other and share our strengths in different areas of expertise. Our different ways of thinking and different approaches to providing healthcare create an enriched system of learning, collaborating, innovating, and sharing of culture.

As I was teaching and beginning a new business, my days were mostly filled with one-on-one consultations. I would hear about the desire of many individuals to be more involved in their own healing and that of their loved ones. Their initiative and motivation to have more control over their own health fueled a greater sense of compassion and sympathy in me. I experienced a change in my approach to healing, as I put less emphasis on highly logical and efficiency-based thinking, to a more holistic, nurturing, and caring perspective. I was able to form more meaningful, trusting connections with my clients, which allowed me to provide more support for holistic long-term healing. Additionally, transitioning quickly between speaking Chinese and English, and between different collaborative working styles, became natural.

I also expanded my focus to methods of healing that were still driven by Chinese medicine ideology, but took place outside the clinic and targeted wellbeing in terms of quality of life. I wanted to support those in the community who expressed their initiative to be more involved in their own health and healing. So, I started teaching tai chi classes, and providing additional support and guidance in breathing, meditation, and qi gong techniques, which were based on yin-yang theories of balance. These methods were ones that can be used by anyone at any time, and I saw that Chinese medicine could help not only with treating illness as it arises, but with illness prevention, and with the holistic improvement of one's quality of life.

During my career, I have found that being exposed to many new ways of thinking, approaches to healthcare, and technology, has guided my constant learning. To compile some of these influences and ideas, I created my own personal website, sharing my own philosophies and values. My days are now a combination of discussing new concepts with my colleagues and peers, teaching and practising tai chi and qi gong, reading about and researching new ideas, appreciating art and talent that my clients share with me, and listening to audio books in between everything. This helps me to connect with more like-minded people, to learn from them, and expand my understanding of health concepts.

My journey in Chinese medicine is ongoing. I have found that my background as a healer comprises a holistic perspective, an understanding of the concept of yin-yang balance, and an ability to seek support within my own spirituality. Heart-felt feeling and sympathy bring me greater awareness of ways I can support my clients and community. This awareness creates a force of intention within me to help the community, creating meaning in my work and actions, and projecting from me a willingness to help others.

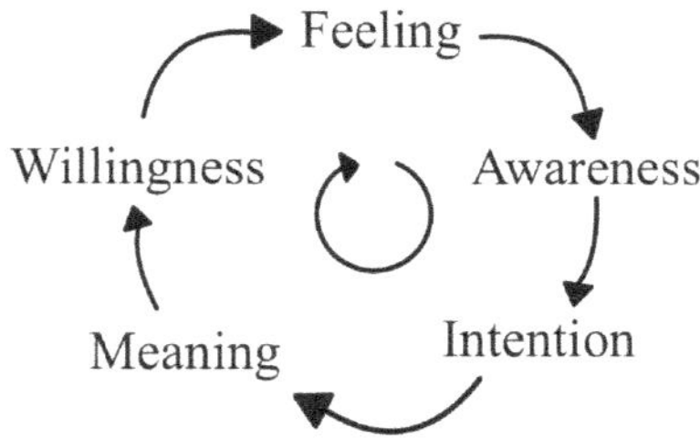

I strive to see connections between traditional Eastern and contemporary modern medicine, and other forms of healing therapies. Through this book, I wish to share my own feelings, knowledge, and views to others, with the hope of building a happy, harmonious, and healthy community together.

NOTE ON PRODUCTION BY PRYOR HOLLIS

I started working at Dr Haisong's Chinese medicine clinic as a personal assistant and administrative staff member in December 2022. By mid-January 2023, a conversation between Dr Haisong and I had begun, about his extensive knowledge of Chinese medicine. That conversation first meandered, but soon picked up pace and direction through 2023, progressing into this very book. Writing for and learning from Dr Haisong has been a great privilege.

Dr Haisong has always been guided by an admirable ambition to share his knowledge with clients and the wider community, with the desire to improve general health and wellbeing for all. So two or three times weekly, while I was working in the clinic, Dr Haisong and I would meet to discuss his ideas for a few chapters' worth of content, sitting across a small table from each other, right behind the clinic's reception desk. The clients arriving and awaiting treatment, and the frequent ringing of the clinic phones, for herbal medicine deliveries, represent the community we wanted to help through the production of this book.

Through hundreds of discussions like these, the structure, content, and purpose of the book formed. At the beginning of the process, I was starting out at university, fresh from a secondary school experience of the intrinsic gendered challenges of being a student of STEM, and following my passions in physics, astrophysics, and French. I had no more knowledge of Chinese medicine than any child of a mixed Chinese-Malaysian-Australian new migrant family might have. I was deeply inspired by these discussions.

Dr Haisong had a way of expressing Chinese medicine philosophy such that I was able to connect with its concepts and practices, even through the often complexly opposing theories of the natural sciences my university lecturers espoused. Through our discussions, we formed a structure for the book, and at the same time, developed a multitude of analogies that best communicated the traditional Chinese medicine concepts, coming from nature, everyday thoughts, and even phenomena explored in particle physics and astrophysics.

Over those many months, I expressed Dr Haisong's philosophy in writing after each of our discussions. Then, with a completed draft, we entered a rigorous process together, of editing and refining, rearranging and restructuring. The final stretch of the process involved the design and formatting of the book - I developed most of the images with AI technology, or by hand-drawing diagrams of concepts Dr Haisong had described to me.

This long process has been an incredible learning experience. I am grateful to have had the opportunity to learn so much from and to work with Dr Haisong, and can only imagine the impact he has on others as a healthcare professional and holistic wellbeing advocate.

PURPOSE

This is a collection of notes on healing, which integrates traditional Eastern and contemporary Western philosophies. Chinese medicine has been practiced for thousands of years, and today, though it is not so commonly practiced everywhere, it is a philosophy constantly deepening, growing, and extending outside of the box. Each chapter explores a new perspective or theory relating to Chinese medicine philosophy and the concepts covered have been inspired by Dr Haisong's own experiences and curiosity. Dr Haisong's colleagues and clients have also collaborated and influenced the ideas throughout the book.

It should be noted that the ideas and concepts in this book should not be taken and implemented in place of any medication or treatment that has been prescribed. Health concerns should still be brought to the attention of the reader's current care team. This book is not designed to inform dramatic changes or ceases to the use of current medication or care programs.

Rather, the purpose of this book is much more about our way of thinking about our health and wellbeing. The philosophies explored within these chapters aim to bring new, creative, and reflective perspectives on healing and wellbeing to the reader, drawing connections between energy flow, mental awareness, and various other concepts and techniques. Central to healing is how we manage our quality of life, which depends on our own conscious choice to improve our health and wellbeing. Our perspectives and approach to healing can be taken into our own hands, with mindfulness and kindness towards ourselves, others, and the environment. We must also learn that we cannot always be in control, and that healing is a process of acceptance and constant growth.

There are many concepts and ideas discussed throughout this book. For the most valuable experience, the reader should maintain a holistic sense of acceptance and appreciation as they encounter these new concepts, or rather, new ways of thinking about healing. The reader should also feel encouraged to draw their own connections between the book's content and their own thoughts, physical health, and emotions. By drawing these connections, the reader can bring about their own personal and meaningful experience, and reflect on how this affects them as individuals, as well as in a social, family, and environmental context.

The holistic model is central to traditional Chinese medicine philosophy. At times, thinking holistically and embracing holistic approaches to healing may seem daunting in its all-encompassing implications. However, to think holistically does not have to be so formal and complex. Holistic thought can simply be about connecting our being with elements of our everyday lives. Throughout this book, we see connections with our immediate environment, our own body parts and organs, the way we sit and stand, and the way we express ourselves through words. These are just some of many examples of how we apply holistic thinking in a tangible and personal way. With time, acceptance, and an open mind, we can see that healthcare takes the shape of elements in our everyday lives, only shone in a different light. This will help to enhance our ability to self-reflect and heal more sustainably.

'I Know You Know', is both the title of this book and the message to you, the reader, that we all have the ability within us to take charge of our own health and wellbeing. As individuals, we each already have the tools to see our lives differently, and the goal of this book is to inspire you to begin on this journey.

DEFINITIONS

Many of the following definitions originate from traditional Chinese medicine philosophy and are referred to frequently throughout the book.

Qi - Energy that regulates the force of life. Qi is present both inside and outside of the body and connects all the elements of the universe.

Meridians - Channels through which qi flows. As qi flows both in and out of the body, meridians exist as a network in the body, and also reach out all through the environment.

Pain - Common sensations of discomfort. These are the sensations that often guide individuals to seek help to improve their health and wellbeing in the first place.

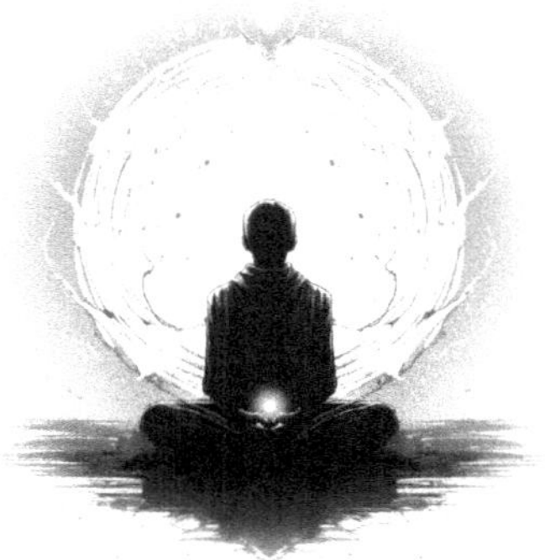

Spirituality - A dimension through which we can understand ourselves - this is different to an understanding that is materialistic, physical, or psychological. Our spirituality involves a sense of both implicit and explicit inner care and self-awareness, and may be expressed through our emotions.

Emotion - Feeling or sensation that comes naturally from within, and can be influenced by our environment, thoughts, beliefs, or values. Emotions often come from our own intuition.

Mind - A conceptual place (linked with the physical brain) that facilitates and generates thoughts, emotions, and responses to different situations. This is not necessarily a physical object.

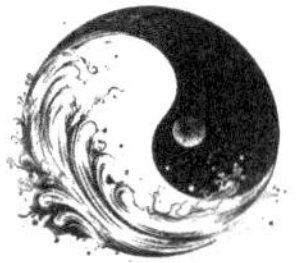

Yin and Yang - The two different directions of the life force. Yin and yang are directly connected, but are opposite in many ways. For example, yin is associated with night-time, the body position of lying down, and femininity, while yang is associated with day-time, the body position of standing up, and masculinity. These are just a few of many examples of the contrast between yin and yang. Throughout this book, we will explore many more contrasts and how they directly affect each other. Most of the time, we seek a balance of yin and yang, as imbalances can pose negative health effects.

Five Elements (wood, fire, earth, metal, and water) - Used to categorise many different aspects in the universe. These categories are expansive, and a few examples include colours, food types, our emotions, and body organs. The elements are closely integrated with nature, and we often seek a balance between the five elements to achieve optimal health. Many holistic healing methods are based on the five elements. Each element is influenced by the other elements, and it is this interaction that creates the flow of energy within us. Consequently, if one element is particularly deficient, it will not effectively generate another element, and this problem can progress.

STRUCTURE OF THE BODY

Part 1

STRUCTURE AND OUR CONTROL

Sometimes, it may feel impossible to pinpoint certain causes of illness or pain, especially when we believe we are regularly making healthy choices. Some individuals describe the phenomenon as feeling as though they have no control over their lives, or rather, that they are in the hands of some higher being.

The truth is, we cannot always know the exact cause of pain, and while we can do research and seek more understanding, we should also be accepting of the fact that there is a limit to our knowledge and control.

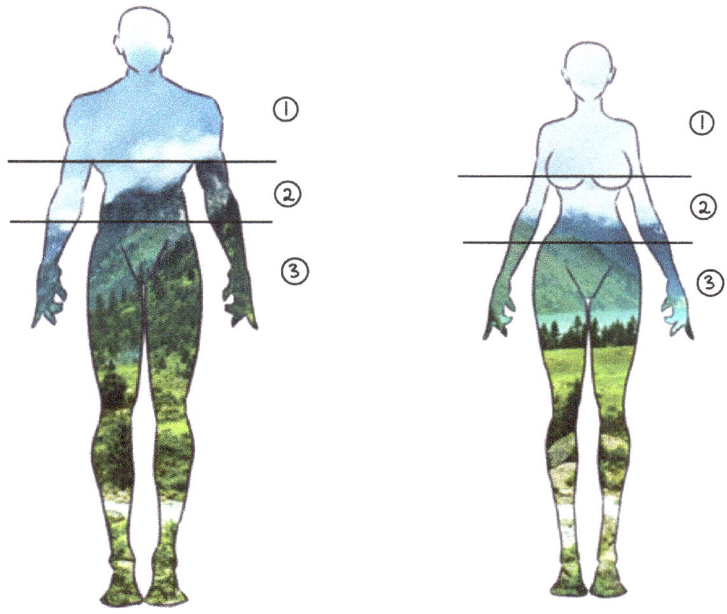

Chinese medicine ideology sees that three different areas of the body correlate with different levels of control we have over our health.

Firstly, we will focus on the area above the diaphragm. This area of the body houses the heart, lungs, and mind, which respectively circulate blood flow, facilitate breathing, and maintain mental stability. These three systems can be argued to influence the most important functions for the body's survival. We might view this area of the body as analogous to a head 'government', governing over the 'society' that is the rest of our body.

Simply because these systems are so critically important and complex, we cannot control their wellbeing and functionality 100% of the time. We can see conceptual connections between our limited knowledge of these systems and that of the sky and outer space. The universe is wide and sparse, containing all that we know and see within it. However, though we can research space with modern technology, we may never truly understand all the systems and processes in the universe. The universe is full of knowledge, yet it will always remain mysterious, giving rise to more questions than answers. Just the same, our own personal mysterious 'universe' lies in this area above our diaphragm.

For example, our brain, breath, and heartbeat, relate to structured and repetitive processes. Our brain repeatedly runs through processes and instructions that keep our body functioning well, our breathing cycles in and out, and our heartbeat regulates blood flow. It is almost as if these systems have pre-coded settings in place, which may be governed by some higher power. The way in which these systems are so perfectly synced to meet our survival needs is difficult to explain, and again indicates that we cannot always have a complete understanding of ourselves and our environment.

A sense of acceptance is key here: we should accept the limit of our understanding, focus less on the sensations of tension or pain, and embrace healing and a greater sense of open-mindedness.

Secondly, we take our attention to the area of the body stretching from the diaphragm to the navel. Most significantly, this area houses the digestive and associated systems, encompassing the sensations of a 'gut feeling' and emotions from within. We can choose what we eat and put into our bodies, which directly affects our health, and by extension, our emotional state. Since we have this greater direct control over our emotional wellbeing, we might refer to this area of the body as the part of us that is most 'human'.

Thirdly, the foundation of our health and wellbeing is dictated by the area of our body below the diaphragm. This area stretches down across our legs and feet. Since this is the lower part of our body, we may identify it as an area of lower importance compared to the first two areas - some may view this area to be in the 'inferior position'. However, this area of the body directly affects our physical structure and stability, acting as a base for all the rest of the body above it. We can run, physically move to different locations, and see the world with this foundation in place. For this reason, we might refer to this area of the body as our own personal 'Earth'.

Without a solid base, or solid 'Earth', we have nowhere to build or grow from. Therefore, it is imperative that we take measures to not only maintain health in this area, but to prevent its damaging or weakening. This part of the body evokes a feeling of gravity, through the feet into the ground, which manifests as warmth due to blood circulation in our feet and joints.

Altogether, these three areas of the body, respectively encompassing essential life systems, the emotional state, and physical foundations, stretch across a spectrum of our indi-vidual control and understanding of ourselves and our health.

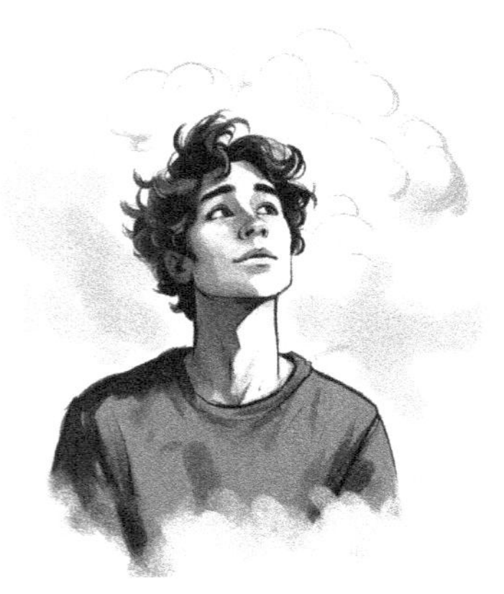

In a sense, we can also see an emerging fourth layer of control, that comes from open-mindedness. Our own willingness to be open to different healing methods and levels of control over our healing invites a crucial layer of control over the effectiveness of our healing journey. This fourth layer weaves within the levels of control from different parts of the body and creates healing energy connections. Many clients coming into the clinic tend to already have concrete ideas around their condition and symptoms, and have suggestions for how best to improve their health. Though having a prior sense of understanding and suggestions for next steps are valued, energy flow is not highly structured, and therefore requires an appreciation of open-mindedness, and to an extent, uncertainty. Energy does not take a specific shape and cannot be structured. Therefore, energy healing methods work best when they are less concrete to accommodate for its free-flowing, unstructured quality. It is important to remain open-minded to be careful not to allow preconceived ideas to take too much of a lead when forming a healing plan.

This open-mindedness welcomes a sense of transparency towards symptoms and healing methods, creating a clearer path of connection between the mind and the body. Thoughts can be expressed more accurately and translated to body movements and motions. In turn, this stronger connection enables us to analyse hidden and expressive pain more deeply, and thus contributes to more effective healing (these different types of pain are discussed in more depth in the chapter, *Types of Pain*, in Part 5 of this book).

For self-reflection ...

What can you do to embrace a sense of open-mindedness towards your symptoms?

Which of the three main areas of the body do you most strongly connect with? What are strategies you can take to connect more deeply with the other areas of the body?

THREE VERTICAL PLANES

We have now seen how we can visualise three areas of the body and how this connects with our levels of control. However, there are many ways in which we can connect with our body and mind. We can also view the body divided into three vertical planes: back, middle, and front. For some, this is easier to visualise, while for others, the structure in the previous chapter makes more sense. The ability to see connections in different ways brings a deeper level of understanding to our bodies and minds.

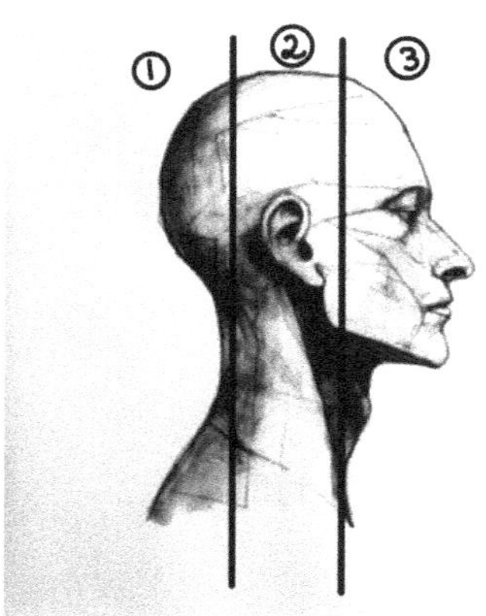

The back plane includes the spine, back muscles, and back part of the brain. The back part of the brain is often known as the 'Animal Brain', governing our survival instincts. It is our basic life control centre, in charge of our ability to breathe, maintain a heartbeat, and strengthen physical balance via the cerebellum and brainstem. We can connect this back plane of the body with the third area of the body specified in the previous chapter (from below the diaphragm to the feet). Both areas function to create a grounded foundation for the rest of the body. We might refer to the back plane of the body as the 'Origin of You' or your 'Truth' as it facilitates our ability to survive on a basic level, or our most 'true' level.

The middle plane includes the ears, jaw, and two large lobes on either side of the brain, and follows the central organs all the way down the body. If you visualise the yin-yang symbol, this middle plane corresponds to the thin S-shape down the centre of the symbol. To balance both sides of yin and yang, this S-shape must be thin and curved. We connect this curvature to the dynamic movement of the body, in the way in which this plane of the body allows us to be flexible, through twisting, turning, and manipulating the body in different ways. This correlates with the central plane acting as a transitional state – a state that is ever-flowing, spirited, and active, and that connects areas between the front, middle, and back planes of the whole body in a flexible manner.

Emotion is the source of our body dynamics. Our emotional state - our source of passion - motivates and drives us to work hard and accomplish goals. Hence, it is evident that this central plane controls our emotional state, and our ability to give meaning to life and create beauty. Beauty, in this context, extends beyond physical or visual beauty. Rather, it is a philosophical understanding of life as an entity of growth and open-mindedness, which allows for opportunities to be presented to us, and appreciation within us. In this way, we may draw a connection between the central plane of the body and the second area of the body outlined in the previous chapter (from the top of the diaphragm to the navel). Both areas are deeply connected to our emotional state.

The front plane includes the front part of the face and brain. This part of the brain controls our learning ability and logical comprehension, specially equipped for managing our cognitive ability, analysing tasks, or computing mathematics. The front plane is also physically developed last, after the back and middle planes. We can visualise this in the way an embryo grows and gradually uncurls, revealing this part of the brain in the later stages of foetal development.

The qualities of kindness and willpower are directly related to the front plane of the body. In order to improve or heal the front plane of the body, one needs to consciously choose to develop their logical and leadership skills. Visually, an analogy of this could be the image of someone physically leaning forward to focus and take initiative in their own development, bowing in the direction of the front plane of their body. Their willingness to lean into their own self-improvement projects kindness towards themselves as they enable growth.

These three vertical planes are also interconnected in many ways. For example, many forms of medicine focus on spinal health, such as chiropractic therapy and physiotherapy. If we analogise the body as a mountain with the peak of the mountain representing the head on the body, the spine forms the pathway or journey up the mountain towards the peak. The essential life systems encompassed in the spine form the life-sustaining trek up the mountain. The middle and front planes of the body, respectively representing centres of transition and logic, form the individual's motivation to engage in their wellbeing. While the back plane provides necessary life support, the middle and front planes combine logic and transition to create emotion and motivation. Overall, the back plane enables the journey up the mountain, the middle plane motivates the perseverance throughout the journey, and the front plane gives meaning to the journey. The *Neijing Tu* diagram, on the following page, is believed to have originated during the Qing dynasty, and depicts this analogy.

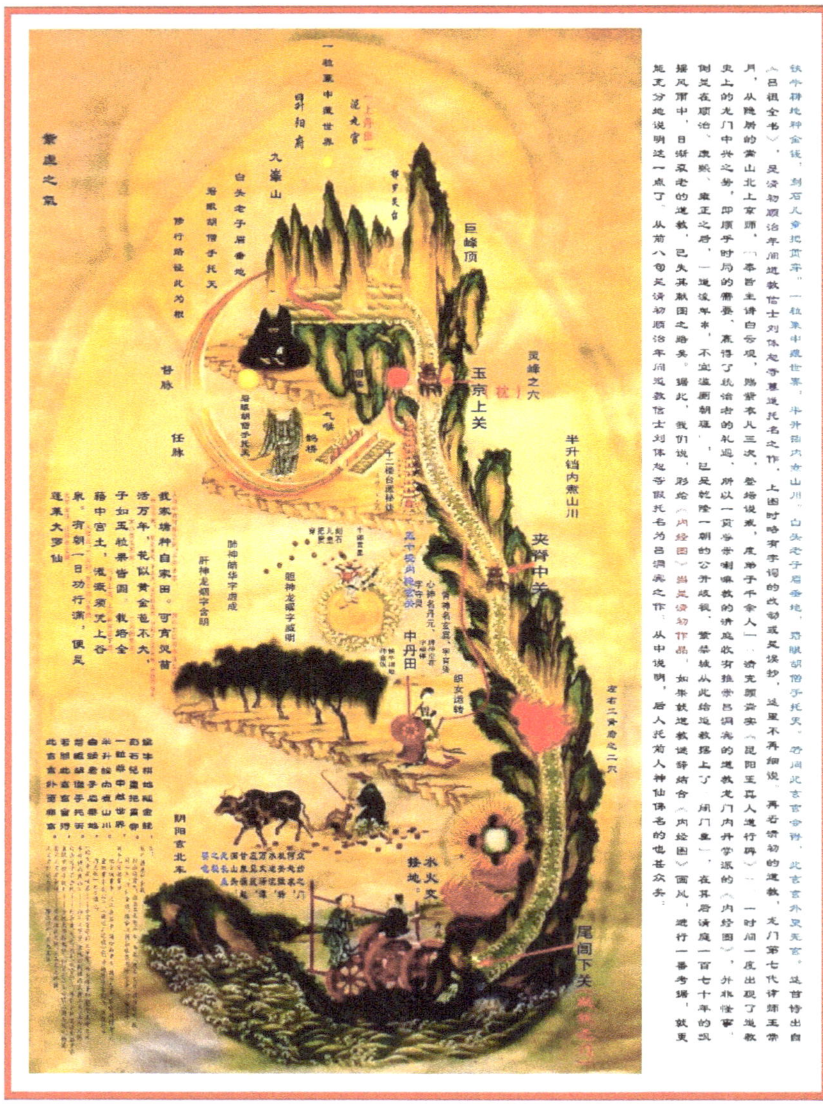

Neijing Tu ('Inner Landscape Diagram') from the Huangting Jing ('Yellow Scripture'). This diagram comes from the Qing Dynasty and represents the human body, depicting the concept of yin and yang balance and qi flow within the body.

Reninger, E. (2021) Neijing Tu, elizabeth-reninger.com. Available at: https://elizabeth-reninger.com/practice-notes-at-the-gym/neijing-tu-large/.

There are steps that can be taken to improve or heal each of the three planes. The back plane can be strengthened by sitting upright to evoke a sense of readiness within. It is also important to train balance and elasticity through the lower legs, back, and spine.

The middle plan can be strengthened through twisting and rotating motions to allow for more transitional freedom. We should also focus on the appreciation of beauty, that is, conceptual beauty. This may be through acts of gratitude or mindfulness. For example, one could simply choose to consume food with a feeling of thanks rather than thought-lessly chewing with abrupt and jarring motions. Often, we find ourselves eating whilst performing other tasks, like working or watching something on the television. These activities are distracting and make it difficult to hone in on the appreciation of beauty in the present.

The front plane can be strengthened through the develop-ment of self-confidence, active use of facial expressions, and monitoring of breathing rhythms. Additionally, we should take initiative to be kind to others and ourselves. Kindness is shared - what comes around, goes around too.

For self-reflection ...

After being introduced to these two different structures in which the body is divided into three, which interpretation most connects with you? Three vertical planes or three horizontal layers?

What type of physical motions can you include in your daily routine to strengthen connection between all three of the vertical planes of your body?

SIX STEPS

Let us add another interpretation of body structure to your repertoire. Learning about new ways of thinking of the body and mind can be a challenge, but the more we embrace new concepts, the more connections we can make within ourselves and with the environment, and thus the more we can do to develop our health and wellbeing.

Moving upward through the body, we can also recognize six 'steps' or parts of the body that are connected. This division of the body dates back to the ancient development of trigrams. Trigrams involved combinations of sticks and stones to create meaning, similar to how a computer uses the digits 1 and 0 in a code.

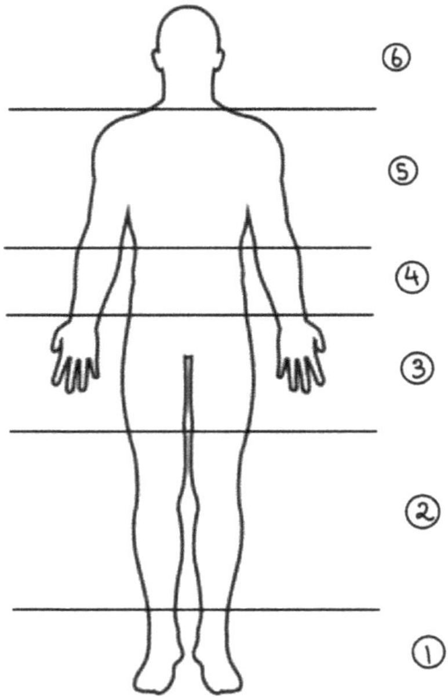

1. Feet and ankles
2. Calves and knees
3. Thighs and hips
4. Abdomen, lower back and stomach
5. Chest, upper back and shoulders
6. Neck and head

A holistic medicine view focuses on the centres of the body. Therefore, although all six units of the body are important, units 2 and 5 tend to attract the most effort and focus for healing purposes.

Furthermore, we can see that there is connection between the upper and lower part of the body, in the way that we can focus on one area to heal the other. Thus, these units can be grouped into pairs, where the strengthening or healing of one part of the pair can help to support the other of the pair. The pairs are 1 and 4, 2 and 5, and 3 and 6. For instance, the healing of unit 3 would support the healing of unit 6. In this way, there is more than one way to target healing within certain steps of the body. This concept of linking the upper and lower body is an example of the interaction between opposing, yet interlinked, yin and yang energies in the body.

In contemporary medicine, there tends to be a strong focus on the health issue at hand, and often, healing plans are made to pinpoint the areas being affected or the areas in which symptoms are present, without much consideration of the linked areas of the body. Chinese medicine, also known as energy medicine, involves the meridian network, with central concepts of yin and yang. This is what drives the connection between the six main areas of the body. For example, in the first pairing, the feet are mostly horizontally oriented in structure, which is a direction closely linked to yin. Conversely, the ankles are a combination of vertical and horizontal components, involving both yin and yang energies. This combination encourages a greater balance of yin and yang.

These pairings also connect with other areas of the body. The feet, for instance, resemble the shape of a kidney, and are thus connected with the kidney via meridians. This means that we can holistically care for the kidney by focusing on healing the feet. Rather than just one part of the body dedicated to all the healing in the body, multiple parts, connected through meridians, can work together in a holistic manner, promoting more effective healing.

In Chinese medicine, the ability to improve health from areas of the body more distant from the area in which symptoms are present, means that we can reveal areas of hidden pain or discomfort. As a result, we can engage in a more comprehensive and sustainable way of healing, instead of solely focusing on one area where expressive pain or discomfort is present (note that the concepts of expressive and hidden pain are detailed later in the chapter, *Types of Pain* in Part 5 of this book).

The complex concept of linking different body parts and meridian pathways is central in Chinese medicine. At first glance, it may be difficult to grasp completely, but as understanding builds, our approach to healing grows much more holistic and effective.

For self-reflection ...

Reflect on injuries or pain you have experienced frequently in the past. Which other part of the body is connected with this area of the body according to the six steps?

How might you balance the process of healing between these two partnered areas to prevent pain in future?

SKIN TO BONE LEVELS

Acupuncture is one of the most common Chinese medicine treatments. When treating with acupuncture, practitioners not only have to think about which areas of the body needles should be placed to best support the body, but also which layers in the skin provide the healthiest qi. This brings us to think about the layers in the skin and how each layer can interact with different parts of the body and our health.

There are five prominent layers in Chinese medicine, starting from the top layer of the skin and moving down to the bone. Each layer is also closely associated with certain organs in the body, listed as follows.

1. Skin and lungs
2. Blood vessels and heart
3. Muscle/soft tissue and spleen/digestive system
4. Tendons and liver
5. Bones and kidneys

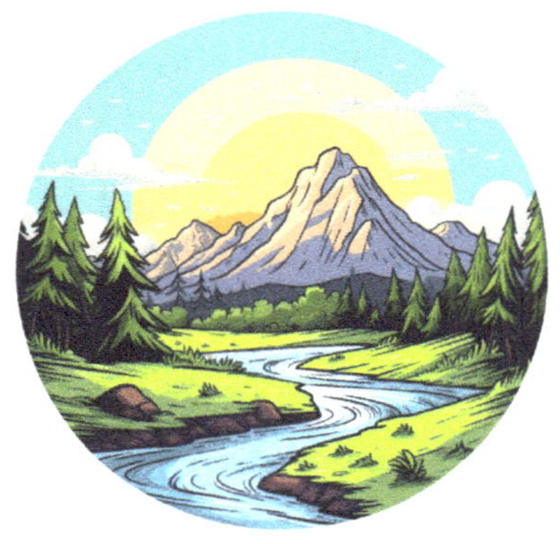

Furthermore, there are important links between each adjacent layer. When these links are strong and healthy, the layers function like a coordinated ecosystem.

The skin and blood vessel layers are connected through the concept of opening and closing of the body. We may see this through the opening and closing of the pores, for example. This connection is directly affected by changes to an environment's temperature. For instance, we may experience goose bumps in cold temperatures (closing of the body) or sweat and perspiration in warm temperatures (opening of the body). The skin-blood vessel connection facilitates the moisturisation and drying of the body.

The blood vessels and soft tissue layers connect through sensations from pressure. Nerves are found all over the body, but the nerves in this layer are particularly prominent. Thus, we may see nerve function affected at this level, and this is usually where acupuncture treatment takes places.

The soft tissue and tendon layers are connected through thin connective tissue, called fascia. Tightened fascia can produce a deep aching pain. Fascia connect through the whole body, and unite the different layers by grouping, holding, and filling up the layers. They also act as connections that can distribute tension across the skin-to-bone layers.

The tendon and bone layers interact with each other through fluid and structure, which hold moisture and allow for movement between the two tougher layers. It is important to have this harmony of hard and soft elements through the fluid and disks to cushion hard impacts that are projected through to this deeper level.

It is important to remember that Chinese medicine focuses on centres of healing. Since there are five skin-to-bone layers, we should focus more on the central third layer (muscle and soft tissue layer) as the most crucial bridge between all the layers. We see in elderly individuals, that as muscle and soft tissue shrink and weaken over time, symptoms such as connective issues start to arise due to the lack of bridging between the five layers. The central muscle and soft tissue layer hold great importance.

By grouping together adjacent layers, we can also see an upper layer (comprising the skin and blood vessels) and a lower layer (comprising the tendons and bones) on either side of the middle layer (muscles/soft tissue). The connection between the upper and middle layers is the place of genuine, healing qi. This is why acupuncture treatment usually remains in this soft tissue layer, where naturally healing qi can be easily accessed and its flow can be redirected. The connection between the lower and middle layers allow for rotational physical movements. We see this connective layer accessed in healing through tai chi training. The practice of tai chi reawakens the rotative ability through our body, whilst maintaining a focus on mindfulness and appreciation of beauty and nature.

These upper and lower layers and their relationships with the middle layer project two significant parts of general treatment in Chinese medicine. The first part is passive treatment, involving treatment that is directly provided to the patient. This includes acupuncture, massage, and herbal medicine. The second part is active treatment, involving the patient's own initiative to heal through movement. This includes the practice of tai chi, mindfulness, or yoga, for example.

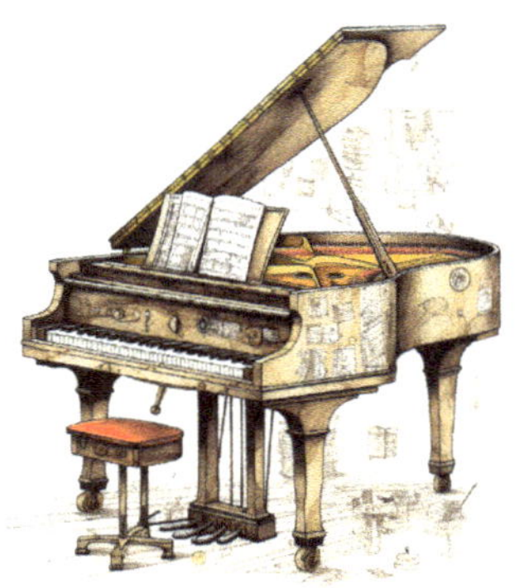

Not only do we see the five individual layers and how they interact with the body, but also how they work together as one mechanism – a mechanism through which we can heal holistically and with care. An analogy for this might be a chord harmony played on a piano. The harmony is distributed across the notes in the chord and the beautiful sound we hear is the culmination of all the pitches. The frequency of the pitch we hear may also correlate to a frequency of energy – much like the mericians that stretch through the layers of the body.

Contemporary medicine focuses on nine main body systems, such as the skeletal system or cardiovascular system. In most cases, symptoms are attributed to different systems, and these systems are analysed independently. In contrast, Chinese medicine sees the body systems to be more interconnected. The interactions in the skin-to-bone layers are one way of interpreting this. Interconnected systems maximise our ability to heal by utilising all the functions available across all systems. For example, if we apply heat to the top layer of skin, it will be transferred down through the lower layers, influencing each layer, down to the bones. This means that we can support deeper layers at a distance, working from the surface of the skin. This is a safer yet practical method of healing.

For self-reflection …

There are examples of harmony, like the harmony we see between the skin-to-bone levels, all around us. What moments of harmony do you experience during your day? How can you take more notice of different aspects in your life coming together in harmony?

POSTURE AND BODY LANGUAGE

Understanding posture and body language is a major part of Chinese medicine ideology. All non-verbal indicators, such as gestures, posture, tone of voice, and amount of eye contact, all send strong messages to those around you. They can put people at ease, build trust, and draw others toward you. Alternatively, they can also offend, confuse, or undermine what you are trying to convey. Appropriate body language and posture help others gain a better understanding of the overall situation, and can thus influence the content of a conversation or a person's voice intonation. Not only are body language and posture important in conversation with others, but also for one's own health.

The front of a person's body not only receives information around them, but also provides information about one's own physical health and wellbeing. The front of the body takes on the full load of the world around them, which is why it is so important to look after your body with nourishing foods, exercise, and mental health consciousness. It is important we also regularly detox the front of the body to remove energy blocks that may be negatively impacting deeper systems in the body.

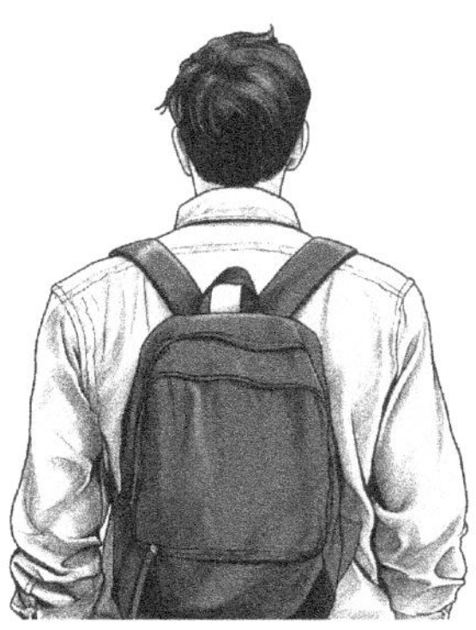

In general, the back of one's body is much safer than the front as you do not need to present it to the world at all times as you would the front of the body. However, it is still useful to take care of the back of the body when relieving pressure from stress or other mental challenges. Through positive body language and posture, you can strive for overall health, wellbeing, happiness, and harmony.

In the context of healthcare and wellbeing, we can often identify the most dominant elements of the five elements of Chinese medicine from one's body posture or body language. Understanding the dominant elements is usually very useful for identifying illness and thus choosing the best routes for healing.

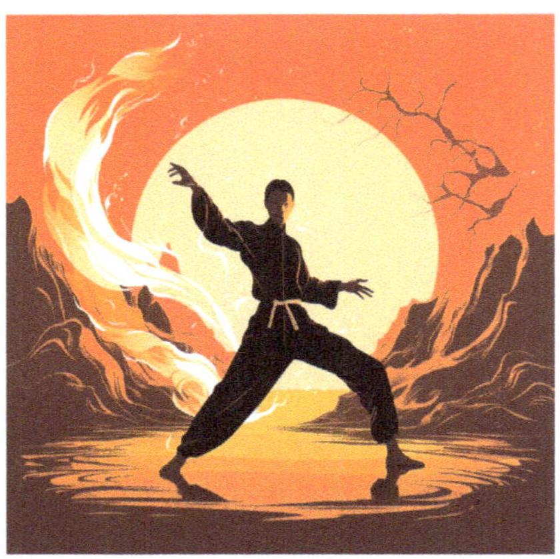

There are two contexts in which we can see dominant elements. The first is when we are relatively healthy. A relatively healthy fire element might be seen through light, quick, and energised movements.

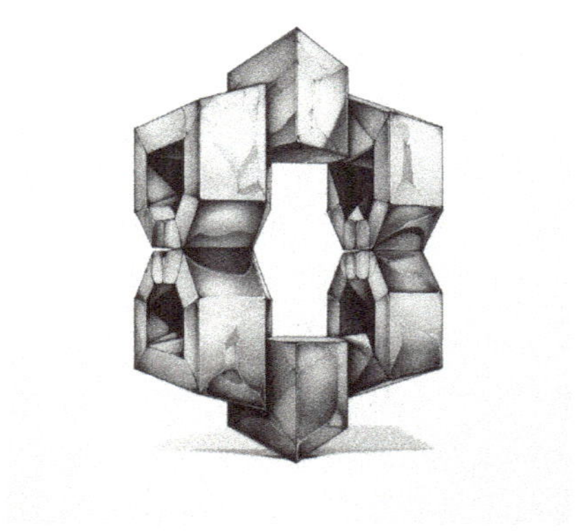

A relatively healthy metal element means that we regulate our posture well, and perform graceful movements with the feeling of peace.

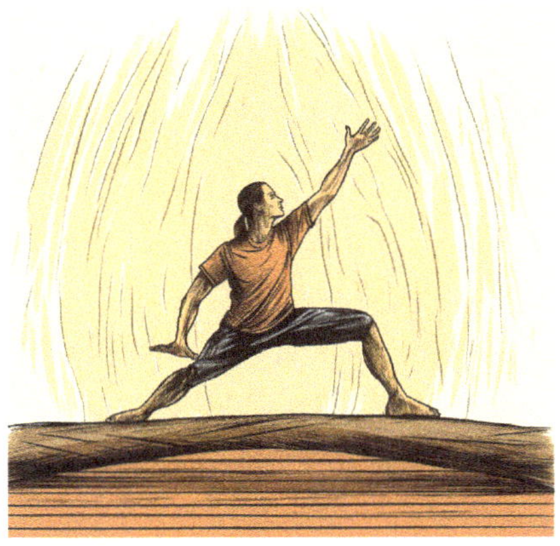

The wood element is associated with upright body posture, good flexibility, and physical extension.

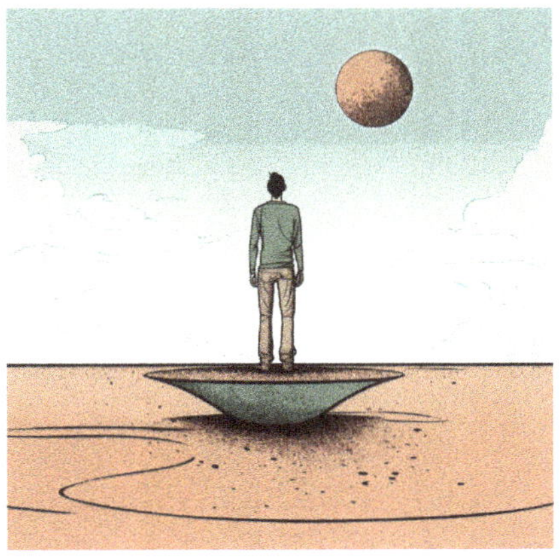

The earth element signifies a solid and stable stance, evoking a feeling that you can depend on your posture and position to remain stable in future.

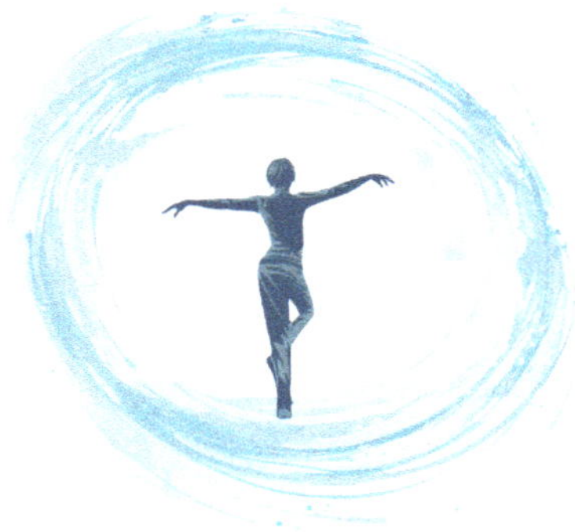

The water element is associated with feelings and sensations of smoothness, gentleness, and flow.

The second context is from the point of view of imbalance between the elements. When the fire element is overpowered, we may experience over-activeness, reactivity, or random changes in our body's dynamics. The imbalanced metal element may create rigidity, unchangeability, or the feeling of being closed-off. The imbalanced wood element may create oblique angles in our body's positions, or a sense of over-rectification. This means that the body overcompensates for injury, sometimes creating over-flexibility in our joints. The imbalanced Earth element may induce heaviness, dull movements, or slumped, overly relaxed body positions. The imbalanced water element may form floppy body positions, or create the feelings of sinking or being driven into the ground, like thick mud as opposed to flowing water.

For self-reflection ...

Which element characteristics most align with your physical movements? Which element characteristics are furthest from your physical movements?

What are some simple, daily exercises or activities you can do to create a better balance between the elements through your physical movements?

HORIZONTAL LAYERS OF THE FACE AND HEAD

The face is usually the first thing we see of someone. It gives us an immediate sense of understanding of a person – we can recognise elements that represent their emotions, which link with their wellbeing and degree of healthy energy flow. Since the face encompasses the nose, eyes, mouth, and ears, which are all linked to the five senses, it also holds great importance in the way that it allows us to receive information from the outside world through our senses.

Additionally, as individuals, we tend to guide our physical movements with the face, as we have to turn to see where we are going and analyse our surroundings. We can see that the face has a strong influence on our physical control, as well as the ability to influence others through our facial responses to the environment. For this reason, when both new or returning clients come into the clinic, often their face is the most immediate, direct way of learning about their current state of mind and wellbeing.

In a previous chapter, *Three Vertical Planes*, we discussed the three vertical planes from the front part of the face through the back part of the head and neck, and how these areas have different associated functions. In this chapter, we will focus on three horizontal layers of the face and head area.

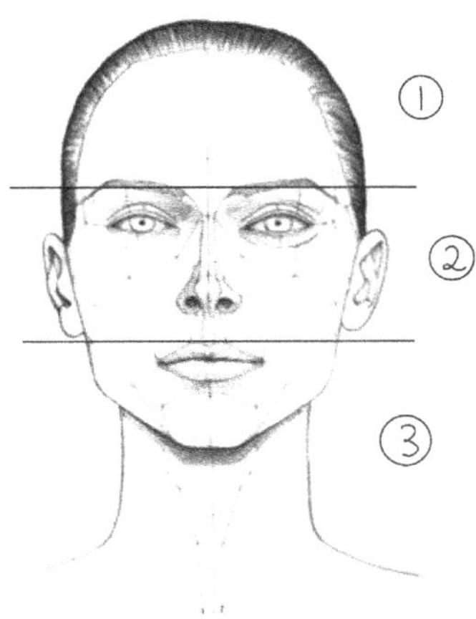

The top layer is from the top of the head to the eyebrow line. This area represents the past, storing past knowledge.

The middle layer is from the eyes to just above the top lip, and includes the ears. This area represents the present and is where we process senses that directly influence our present moment, including our sight, hearing, and smell.

The lower layer extends from the mouth to the bottom of the chin, representing the future. Our thoughts form in our mind and transmit instruction to our mouth – this area is the last area to project expression. It is also this area that allows us to communicate verbally with others, and is what invites others to respond to us. In this way, this area greatly influences the future. The mouth is also where we take in food and nutrients. It takes some time before the food we consume can convert into nutrients and energy. Thus, this is again associated with the future. We can see this in the common example of a diet - diets are often long-term solutions for gradual improvement to health, and we only see the results in the future.

In a sense, our whole body's existence is determined by the past. We are here as the consequence of decisions and circumstances that have taken place in the past. It is therefore very easy to dwell in the past, and much more difficult to live in the present, or even look towards the future.

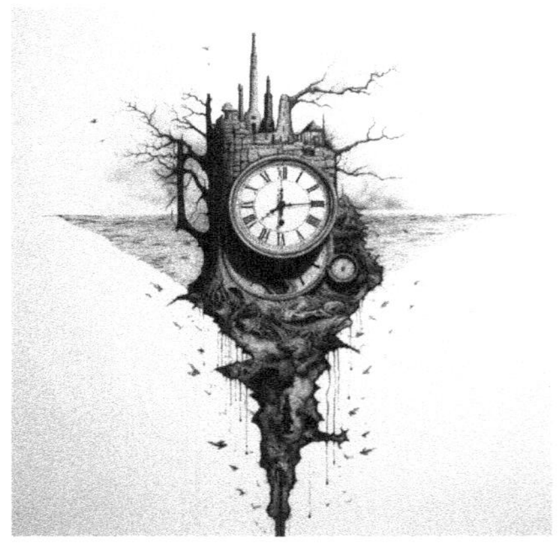

From this perspective, we can see that aspects of life that are associated with having power, leadership, or dominance, represent the past. Aspects of life that are unclear, we are unsure of, or are highly inclined to change, represent the present. And finally, aspects of life that are weaker, hidden, or appear to have great potential, represent the future. This is echoed in the divisions in the body described earlier in this chapter. The top layer (head to eyebrow) is where we make decisions about where our power goes. The middle layer (eyes to the top lip) is where many of our senses lie, including our eyes, nose, and ears, which all perceive and take in our present surroundings. The lower layer (mouth to chin) pro-vides us ways of responding to our environment, and taking in food and nutrients.

This interpretation reveals the importance of caring for our relatively weak points, which are closely linked to the future. By working with our weakest points, we build up our strength to move into the future. From this, we can also see the great importance of caring for our senior and elderly members of the community. As we grow in age, we become physically weaker, but our knowledge continues to grow, and can have a profound impact on the future of our society.

For self-reflection …

Reflect on your most pressing or regular concerns and worries … are these associated with the past, present, or future? Which of the three areas of the head is linked to this time frame?

What are things that you do during the day that prepare you for better health and wellbeing in the future?

INTERACTION BETWEEN THE FACE AND ABDOMEN

Sometimes, when clients come into the clinic, they have already done research on the symptoms they are experiencing and have identified ways through which they can improve their health. Often, clients talk about research they have found on gut health and its connection with brain health. This brings to mind conceptual connections with yin-yang philosophy.

The face and abdomen are the two areas of the body that respond most to our surroundings and express emotion. Our face expresses emotion through facial expression, and our abdomen expresses emotion through sensations such as 'gut feeling' or tension.

The abdomen area can also be divided into smaller areas. The top part contains the heart, the middle layer contains the digestive system, and the lower layer contains the kidneys. Structurally speaking, the liver is located on the right side of the body. However, the liver is represented on the left side of the abdomen area, while the right side of the abdomen area represents the lungs.

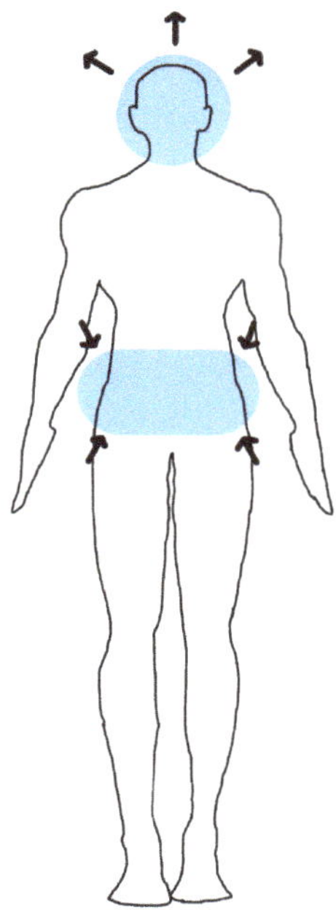

This seemingly swapped representation may be explained by the general direction of energy flow in the body. A healthy body has qi that flows in a circular direction so that some energy flows upwards through some organs and downwards through others. For example, the liver represents the wood element, and wood generally grows upwards. Therefore, the energy flows upward through the liver. Conversely, the lungs correspond to the metal element and the sky whose energy is projected downwards through rain and precipitation. Therefore, the energy flows downward through the lungs. Here, we can see a strong connection between the human body, the flow of qi and the environment.

Furthermore, the face and abdomen are associated with yin and yang qualities. The face, which is outwardly expressive is associated with yang, while the more concealed, private abdomen is associated with yin. It is important that we look after both areas to achieve a balance of yin and yang. Further, if one of these areas is affected by illness, looking after solely the area affected would be insufficient - both areas should be cared for. For example, if an individual suffers from stomach issues, the head area should also be treated to maintain balance. These two areas are highly interactive and share mutual benefits, so we should always consider the wellbeing of both areas simultaneously. Additionally, it has been found that bacteria in the abdomen can directly link to emotions, thought, and decision-making.

In the previous chapter, *Horizontal Layers of the Face and Head*, we discussed how different parts of the body represent the past, present, and future. In this context, interactions with the face represent the past and interactions with the abdomen represent the future (the abdomen is much more hidden than the face). With this association, it becomes clear that while the face is much more visible, we should also remember to listen to our abdomen, which is more closely related to our future health.

For self-reflection ...

Would you consider yourself a highly expressive person? Or do you more often find yourself concealing your emotions?

If you find yourself connecting more with expression outwards or within, try to draw more attention towards the other type of expression during moments of mindfulness.

MIND CONNECTION WITH THE PHYSICAL

Part 2

MIND, THOUGHT, AND MOVEMENT

When we meet new people, before having even talked to them, the first thing we notice is usually their body posture and general movement. Likewise, this is often the first thing we notice about clients coming into the clinic for the first time. The mind is concealed within us, and it is body movements that can express these. Our thoughts form the connection between our mind and body movements.

The thoughts within us dictate both our physical movements and everyday functions. In this context, healing takes place when we mend, develop, and strengthen the connection between our mind and our variety of movement. We cannot survive without life-essential movements, such as breathing, gut movements, or maintaining a level heartbeat. Thankfully, we do not need to put much conscious thought into forcing these fundamental actions – they usually happen naturally.

Varying movement is another essential part of health. It not only helps us to achieve complex tasks, but provides us the freedom to express emotion and access creativity within ourselves. With conscious thought, we can decide to manipulate our body in certain ways. Examples of varying movement that require more awareness include dance movements, trying a new sport, or learning an instrument.

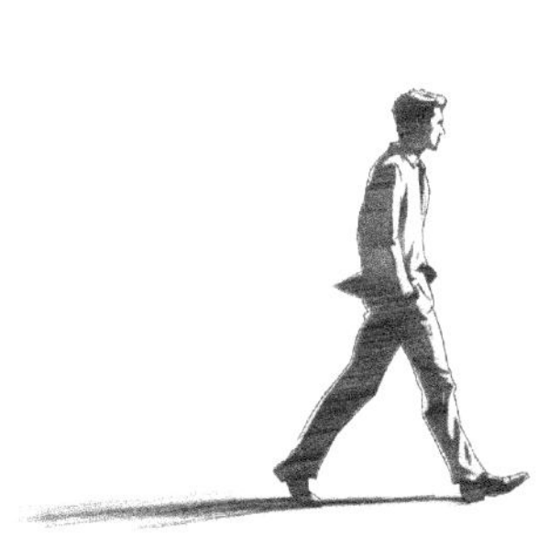

Let us discuss a more in-depth example. An individual may aim to increase the distance they walk every day from 5 km to 8 km. In terms of the variety of movement, this is an example of one-dimensional growth. The individual is only aiming to increase their distance travelled, and no other aspects or associated skills. A more multidimensional goal might be to engage in some new type of physical movement, much different to walking.

Another example of connecting mind with thought, is through varying our familiar movement patterns. Rather than walking normally, we may walk with bent knees and a lower stance, in a sideways motion, with a leg-crossing motion, or with the same arm and leg synchronised. These unfamiliar motions create and strengthen new pathways in the mind.

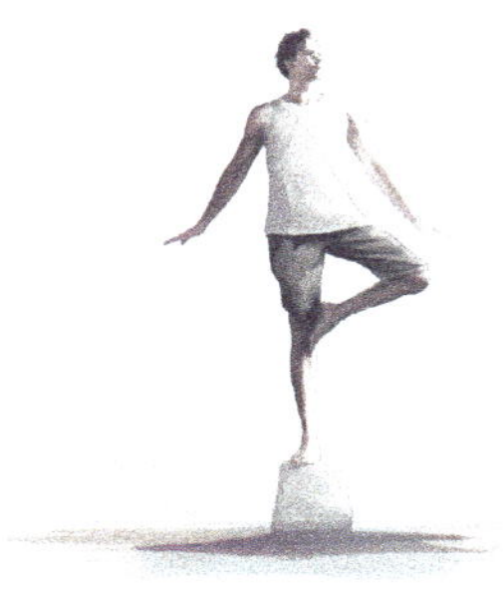

We can vary a standing position by standing on one leg or shifting our weight to the front of our toes, for example.

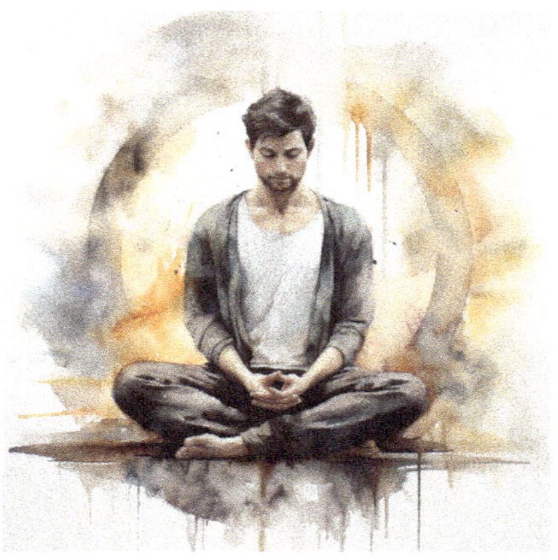

When sitting, we can try squatting, kneeling, cross the legs, or having both legs positioned on one side of the body.

When lying down, we might place one hand in front of us and one hand behind our back, hold our weight forward, keep our feet together, or position ourselves in a face-down orientation. Another lying-down position that introduces more variation is where the individual lies on their back with their legs bent and hips turned- out so that the feet are touching – this is sometimes called the 'frog' yoga position. The hands may rest in a prayer position to help centre the mind and breathing. Unfamiliar movements and positions send different, new signals to our mind, creating harmony as connection between the mind, body, and movement, grows.

To improve their ability to express emotion, connect with others, and grow in creativity, individuals should embrace varied types of movement, which is achievable through open-mindedness, patience, and willpower.

For self-reflection …

Take note of the physical movements you do during your daily activities … are there certain movements you do frequently?

What new activities or physical movements can you practice to strengthen your body-mind connection?

ONE MECHANISM: MIND, BODY, AND BREATH

We hear about the importance of breathing in a lot of activities related to health and wellbeing … in meditation, yoga, team sports, and during many moments of stress, for example. At times, we hear so much about breathing that we can sometimes lose touch with why exactly it is important. In Chinese medicine, we see breathing as another connection between our mind and body. Breathing grounds us in the present moment, and the more mindful we are about our breathing, the more cohesively our body works as a healthy system.

The mind controls thoughts and our mental stability, and the body maintains posture and spatial awareness. During the healing process, it is normal for the mind to wander to other external areas of focus. However, true, meaningful healing cannot really commence until a connection between the mind and body is established. In a sense, the mind's focus is what primarily encourages healing to progress effectively.

Calm breathing that projects through the whole body can be a powerful avenue of connection between the mind and body. A simple example is in a common acupuncture treatment. To allow a healthy flow of qi through the body via acupoints, the patient should focus on the acupoints by

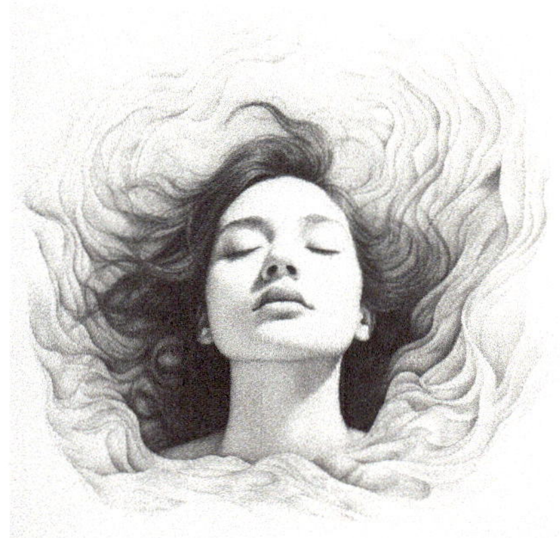

breathing and drawing focus, calmly, to their points of pain. A wondering or distracted mind will only take away from the acupuncture treatment and the progress of healing.

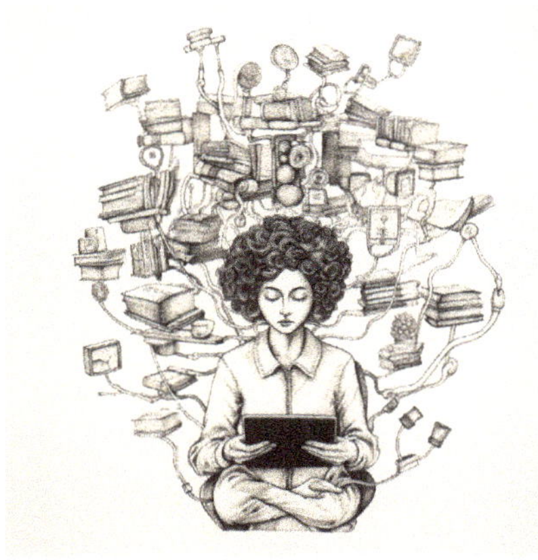

This concept of drawing focus to one place is also relevant in activities that might allow for multi-tasking. The process of multi-tasking, or the ability to perform multiple tasks at once, is actually physically impossible. When we multi-task, we are rapidly switching between two activities, causing distress on the mind as we swap between sometimes completely different trains of thought. The best way of completing tasks, is by focusing on one activity at a time, just like the focus we should have on our healing when we most need it.

Additionally, we can obtain greater mind-body connection by paying attention to the direction of our breath. Positive energy from the environment works from the outside-in, while our mind works from within our bodies and projects outwards. Breathing involves inhaling and exhaling in directions both outside-in and inside-out. With an inhale we draw in the positive energy in our environment, and with an exhale, we release the energy built up in our mind from thought.

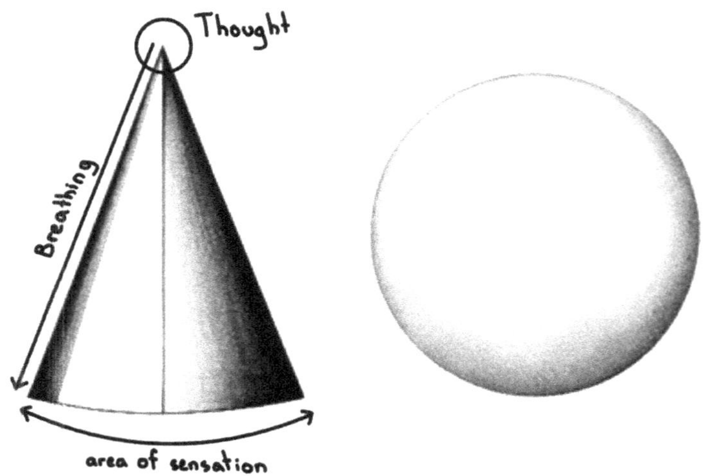

We can also visualise the mind-body-breath connection in a drawing. Thoughts can be represented by dots or small circles on a page. Breathing is represented by lines drawing out from the dots, and the body sensations form the base of the 3-dimensional shape that forms. In this way, the dot (thought) connects via a line (breath), and forms an area of sensation (body). As this process repeats in the same area, we might see that a cone forms, and over time, a complete sphere will form. Read on to the next chapter, *Shapes*, where we explain more about the energy and health benefits of conceptual spheres.

For self-reflection ...

During what activities or specific periods of time do you find yourself feeling the most anxious, stressed, or out of control?

Notice if your breathing changes during these moments, how can you bring more presence through your breathing?

SHAPES

Everyone has a unique identity. Similarly, objects and materials have identities as well, defined by their physical shapes. If objects did not have defined physical shapes, we would find it quite difficult to separate different objects and see the world with physical clarity. In this way, an object's 'identity' is really just a way of separating and differentiating between different objects.

When clients come into the clinic feeling confused or unstable, this understanding of shapes can bring them some immediate clarity. Chinese medicine philosophy extends this understanding a step further, connecting different energy levels with different shapes.

Our environment is comprised of various shapes and edges, from the objects we see to the physical motions we experience. In Chinese medicine ideology, shapes and edges project meaning, help us to develop more effective healing processes, and support us in performing everyday activities.

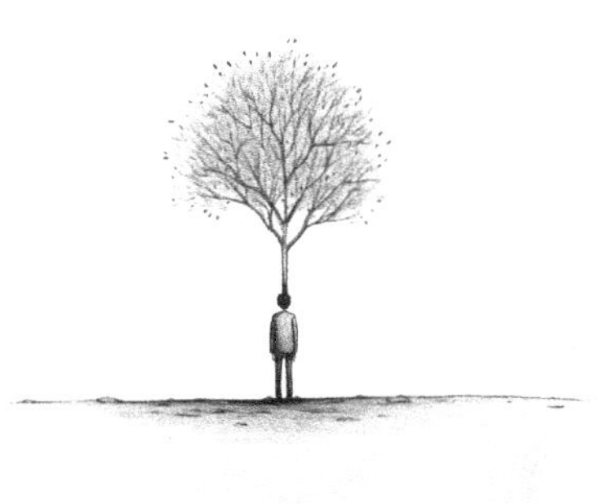

For example, we form an upright tree-like position when we are standing, or a curved and rounded bowl-like shape when we are lying down. When we walk, we form a vertical position that is also moving forwards, much like a breeze, and when we are sitting, we often resemble the stable and unwavering form of a grandfather's clock.

Disturbances to healing may cause imbalance and thus distortion of some of these shapes. Objects with a circular or curved shape represent a sense of harmony. One might connect this with the curved lines in the symbol of yin and yang. The curves are flowing, and form a cycle, rather than an abrupt, concrete end. Rounded, circular shapes and edges represent self-sufficiency, sustainability, and healthy flowing energy.

Angles and sharp edges that we see in the environment correspond with rigidity and a stage of uncertainty. Stress can manifest in these rigid angles, limiting one's ability to relax and breathe comfortably, and thus reducing the progression of healing. Angled, sharp corners and edges represent abruptness and stiffness.

For example, many meditative practices encourage relaxation and the rounding of the arms and posture to allow for more circular breathing and healing relaxation. Feeling physically or mentally tense, or metaphorically 'sharp', can greatly take away from the healing focus of mindfulness practice.

It is important to remember that these shapes are very much conceptual, and only sometimes will take the form of a physical shape. The yin-yang symbol is an example of a physically rounded shape. However, if, for example, imagine an individual had a rather round stomach. This is not necessarily considered 'roundness' as the stomach would still protruding from the body. Rather, it is creating a less healthy edge on the body. In this case, we should note that the structure and position of the whole body should be considered. One might argue that a standing position is not rounded, which is true in the physical form, but someone who is healthy and upright would be able to move around more freely, forming circular, flowing, and rounded movements.

In a practical setting, many clients who have sharp points in their lifestyle find it difficult to adjust their perception and approach to healing. These 'sharp points' may be related financial hardship or old age, for example. In these cases, we should remind ourselves of the various aspects that contribute to life, and that there are ways in which we can continue to thrive and grow beyond certain 'sharp points' we may face on our journey.

For self-reflection ...

What are the prominent 'sharp points' in your journey? Just taking notice of these points brings consciousness and thus roundedness to these aspects of your life.

CONCEPTUAL SPHERES

When clients come to clinic, we always encourage that they try to heal in ways other than receiving treatment. One common way of doing this is through practicing mindfulness. However, sometimes, it can be difficult to find a time of day to dedicate solely to the activity. It is important to remember that mindfulness takes many forms. In Chinese medicine philosophy, we may connect this with the concept of roundedness and circular shapes.

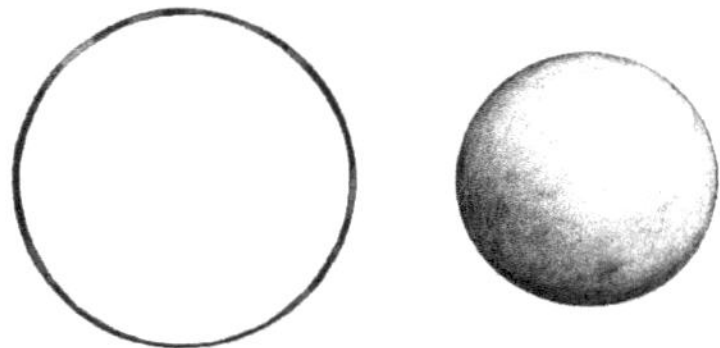

In the previous chapter, *Shapes*, we discussed the value of the circle and other curved shapes as favourable forms of healing and positive energy. The circle itself is two-dimensional, similar to a dot or a line. In this way, the 'conceptual circle' can reach a higher dimension, and with it, a stronger level of healing. The 'conceptual circle' takes the form of a spherical shape. All healing should gradually work towards achieving a spherical state. An individual may experience sensations analogous to a two-dimensional line or dot, as long as their treatment aims to bring them to a spherical state of positive energy and growth over time. We can achieve this by considering a third element, such as reflecting on memories or our own degree of self-awareness, in our daily activities. For example, instead of mindless walking (which is quite two- dimensional), an individual could focus on the purpose in their steps and their goals in the present moment. This creates a structure that connects the physical and the conceptual, promoting rounded energy.

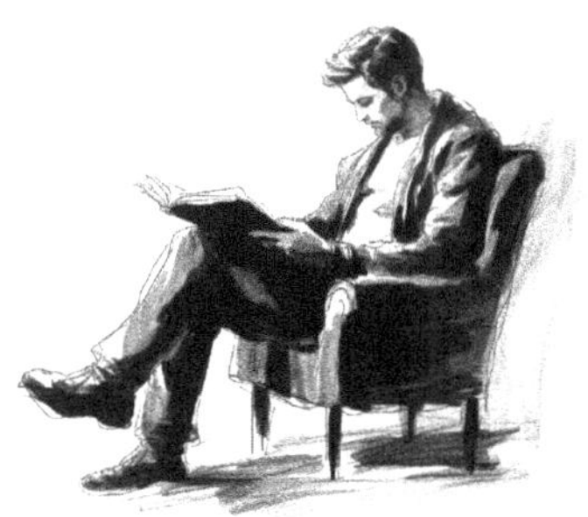

Another example might be as simple as visualising scenes as you read a book. Try to match the emotions you feel as you read with the images and colours that naturally arrive in your mind.

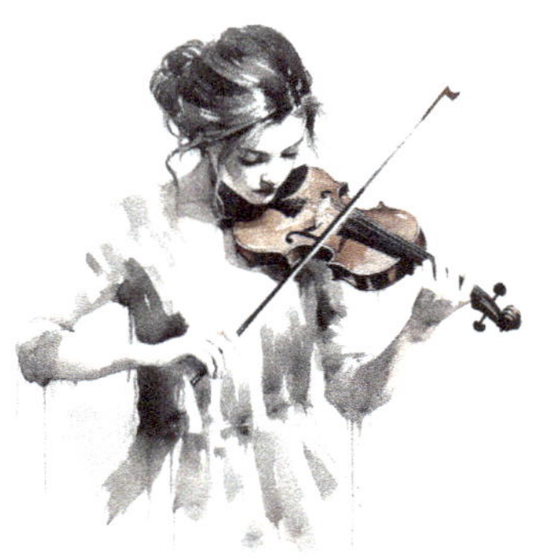

Or, if you play an instrument or sing, you could link a certain past memory to the music. This imagery can act as a source of emotion. Emotion dictates dynamics or volume in a musical piece (i.e. whether parts of the song or instrumental piece are played softly, loudly, fast, or slow). Let a memory guide the feeling of your music, and connect spiritual thought with the physical movement through your hands.

We can also link the spherical, round shape, to the presence of all five elements in Chinese medicine: fire, earth, metal, water, and wood. These five elements are often presented together as a five-point star. As the elements transition into each other, the five points gradually merge into a flowing circle. Therefore, a circular shape may be said to be most healing as it involves a balance and healthy cyclical transition between all five elements. As soon as energy takes a non-spherical or non-rounded shape, only one or two elements are present. For example, a regular pen would likely encompass two main elements, as its shape has two physical end points. The elements in non-rounded shapes tend to be in contrast with each other, though they will still interact with each other. However, if one element is dominant over the other, it will gradually encourage a harmful imbalance of the elements.

With just two elements, we can have many different relationships: fighting, struggling, agreement, or support, for example. Regardless of the type, any form of interaction is in some way good, as it invites the need for a third element's presence, which acts as a moderating element. Therefore, we should employ healing methods that allow for a third element to be brought into the system. The third element is likely to bring greater harmony, by sharing power to the less dominant of the present elements and taking overpowering strength away from the dominating element.

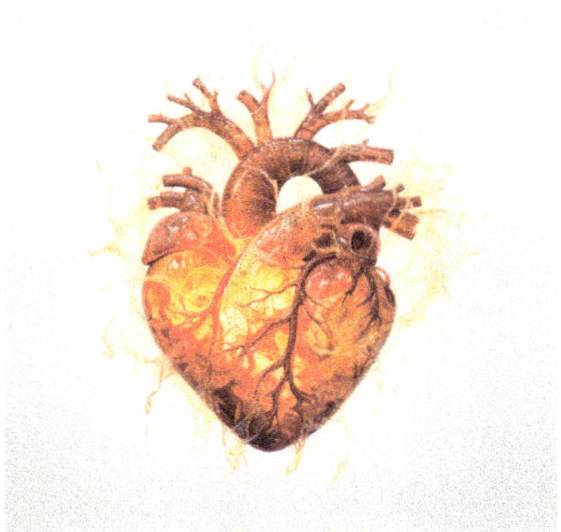

As an example, if someone has extra heat in their heart, then their fire element is likely dominant. This might manifest in symptoms such as overthinking, stress, or disturbed sleep. An immediate thought might be to introduce water to the system by drinking more water, as it opposes the fire element more so than the other elements. However, this may pose too much of an immediate contrast that may shock the system and cause greater damage.

Alternatively, we should bring water into the system through a certain path or amount that is associated with a third element. For example, we may drink water in small amounts, over spaced-out intervals of time during the day, or in a quiet place. These characteristics are typical of the metal element.

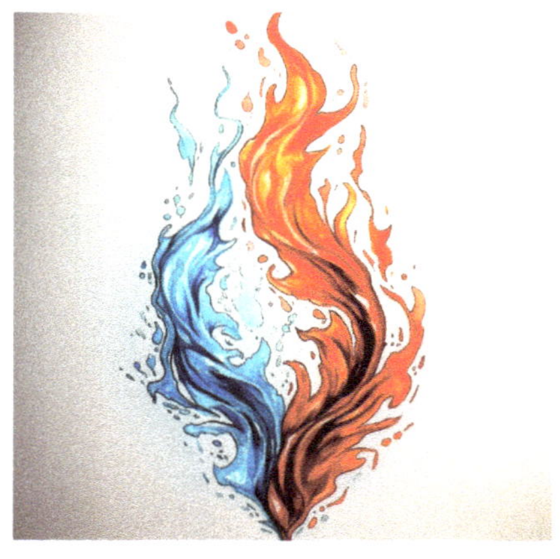

Here, we have introduced metal as a third element, encouraging interaction between the fire and water elements. The role of the third element is to give structure to the healing process, and healing plans should be developed to include the third element's features.

For self-reflection ...

What daily activities often come naturally to you? These are often a good place to start integrating a new level of thought and mindfulness. What emotions or memories can you connect with these activities?

BODY, MIND, AND SPIRITUALITY

After receiving treatment, clients often inquire about what they can do away from the clinic and in their own time to support their healing journey. Some frequent recommendations are related to adjusting lifestyle, diet, or exercise, for example. However, in Chinese medicine, we also consider recommendations related to the body, mind, and spirit.

For instance, if the client's treatment is quite active, frequent, or intensive, we would recommend mind-relaxing activities to balance the physically active component of treatment with a more relaxed mental component of recovery. Conversely, if the client's treatment is minimal and they are in generally good health, we would recommend focusing on mental activity and staying alert and conscious of their surroundings. This may help the client take note of changes in their lifestyle that may affect their health in future.

The body, mind, and spirit interact and influence each other through every thought, movement, and sensation. The body connects with our physical movement and actions, and comprises materials and life energy. The mind connects with our knowledge, ability to problem-solve, life energy, and our consciousness. Spirit brings forth our feelings and beliefs, and comprises our consciousness and presence in the universe. Often, our spirituality is projected through our emotions.

It is imperative that these three aspects work in unison to achieve balance. For example, when the body is physically comfortable, it may feel easy to let the mind and spirit (and thus emotions) relax and wander, to achieve a similar relaxed state. However, to maintain balance, the mind and spirit should remain active and energised. Remaining productive in these areas will prevent an individual from feeling helpless or thoughtless. In the case where thoughts may be very complex or difficult to work through, it is important to employ the spirit and emotions as well in order to avoid overloading the mind. By keeping the mind and spirit challenged, we create balance with the body physically relaxed.

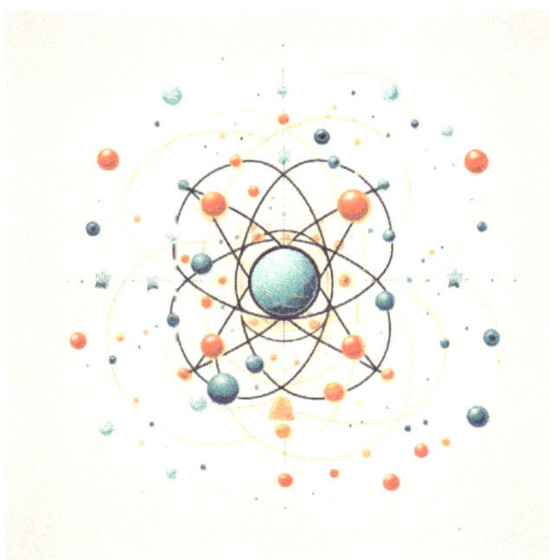

With balance comes the importance of control and stability. Too much energy in one state creates instability. This also relates to many concepts in the natural sciences: the environment naturally tries to share energy rather than store it in one area. In the tiny atoms that make up our universe, there are negative electrons that occupy space around each atom.

Energy is spread across both the atom and its electrons to increase stability. We can also see a similar phenomenon in magnetic fields across our globe, where energy is dispersed between the north and south magnetic poles, for example. To attain this stability, the mind should attempt to embrace beautiful thoughts, encompassing creativity, memories, and positive human qualities. This circulates positive energy throughout the body.

For long-term ongoing pain, harnessing emotions can be powerful. It is important to recognise that emotions are always in transition and are not stagnant, and therefore, it is natural to experience both positive and negative emotions in a cyclical manner. For example, sadness may lead to fear and anxiety, which encourages us to employ critical thought to plan and cope with our anxious feelings. After a plan is formed, there may come a sense of serenity, and then joy, which may then provide the space for an individual to recognise concern again, and the cycle repeats.

We have now discussed the importance of achieving balance between these three aspects - we can also interpret this as interactions between each of them. We can think of this concept as our body positions and physical structure informing how mentally focused we should be. For example, there are many different forms and paces of breathing: deep breaths, short breaths, long sighs, or quick in-takes. Our breathing directly affects our mental and physical state. Holding breath may naturally induce feelings of pressure or stress. This may then create fear, and may connect with the concept of death as we appear not to be breathing at all. If we over-exhale or breathe too rapidly, we might faint or experience blurry vision, affecting our productivity. Therefore, we can develop a highly valuable healing mechanism to regulate our breathing and emotion, by observing and changing the length and frequency of our breaths and remaining conscious of its direct impact on our mental and physical state.

For self-reflection …

When you are feeling stressed, notice any changes in your breathing rhythms. Can you tell if these changes create new feelings within you?

Are there moments during the day when you feel especially mindless or unfeeling? What ideas or emotions can trigger more mind activity during these times?

VISIBILITY OF EMOTIONS

Emotions can be thought of as an atmosphere – they grow, expand, and turn into new emotions. Atmospheres are also wide, expansive, and seemingly uncontrollable. It is difficult to identify the boundaries between different emotions, just as it is difficult to identify where an atmosphere starts and ends.

Emotions are visible in the sense that they are expressed through facial expression, posture, tone of voice, and more. However, they encompass invisible energy, which controls and directly affects how emotions are translated outwards to become visible. It is the connection between being concealed inside to being expressed outwardly, via invisible energy and visible 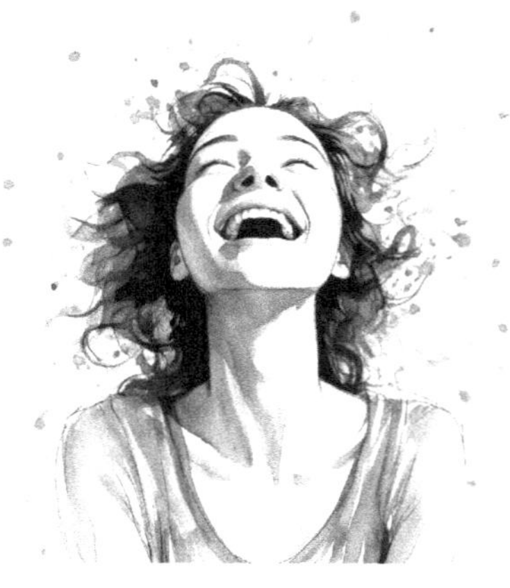 appearance, that creates balance and meaning in our feelings and sensations related to emotions.

We should not ignore or push away our emotions, but try to meet and accept them instead. In some cases, emotions can be so overwhelming that it makes the mental and physical states complex. It can then become difficult to make proper logical decisions or maintain a peaceful, harmonious state.

Additionally, emotions generate new emotions, some of which are beneficial in the moment, and some of which are not. Reiterating from the previous chapter, it is important to remember that emotions are constantly changing and developing from each other.

Individuals should also focus on maintaining balance across the mind, body, and spirit, especially when dealing with very strong emotions. Even though the spirit is the main state in which emotions are formed and controlled, the mind and body should help to manage emotions by employing physical and logical coping mechanisms. One way to do this is to visualise emotions as shapes. This could take any form in the mind: emotions sifting in and out of you, pouring over you, or enveloping you.

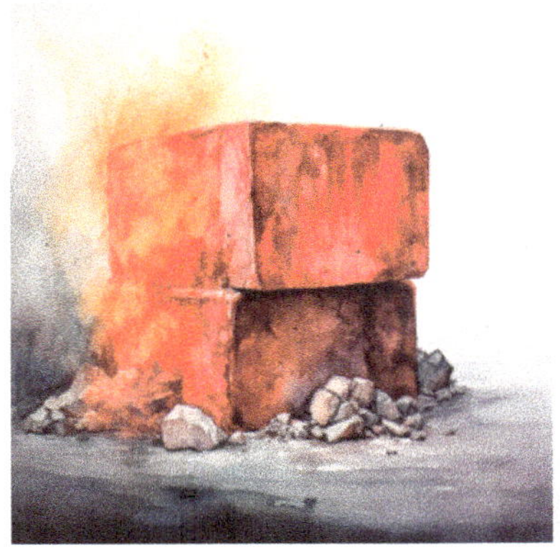 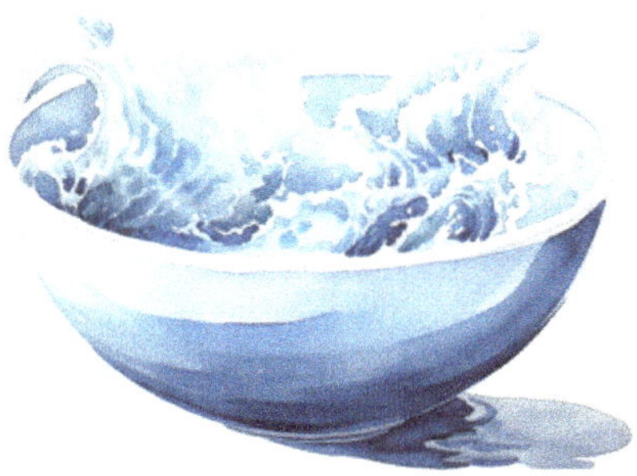

One might envision a chunk of anger, a bowl of sadness, or a container of curiosity. This can help us recognize when and encourage emotions to transition into new emotions through a change of shape or physical representation.

When we materialise our emotions by associating them with physical shapes such as these, we create a powerful healing mechanism. Even our largest and most overwhelming emotions can be projected into these much smaller, more manageable shapes and objects. We describe this process as the 'formless' confining itself into the 'formed'. The emotions encompass energy within the shape they form in our mind.

There are ways of visualising emotions in the physical form other than through shapes and objects. For example, by listening to music or dancing we can translate our emotions into what we hear or the body positions we form.

We would not have balance without the ability to transition the other way as well, from formed to formless. This is a transition sometimes known as 'subliming'. This process brings more energy into the individual, taking in the energy from a distinct form or shape within the surrounding environment. Depending on the situation, this can also have benefits, one being the ability to philosophise on a greater, grander scale, with more energy.

Another way we can visualise the concept of transitioning from the formless to the formed, and vice versa, is through a triangular structure of essence, energy, and spirit. In traditional Chinese medicine, these three elements transfer between other, creating flow and balance. Essence represents blood and physical material, energy represents qi energy and the force of life, and spirit represents one's mentality, mind, and focus. For example, when we age and slow down, our mind becomes stronger and we become wiser. This can be explained as essence transferring into spirituality. That is, physical material transforming into the mind and thoughts.

For self-reflection ...

What physical representations of emotions feel the most natural for you to visualise?

PROJECTING TO THE ENVIRONMENT

Many clients come to the clinic with the understanding that the environment can directly affect our emotions and mental state. However, in Chinese medicine, we often look for balance, and we see that we can also project outwards to the environment with feelings that come from within us. Our emotions dictate what we do and the decisions we make. Therefore, it is important to regulate our emotions and mental health. There are many ways of doing this, and this chapter will hone in on one particularly effective and practical strategy that can be applied anywhere and anytime. This strategy is based on our five senses and our environment.

Sight allows us to receive the most information compared to our other senses. We should focus on five important objects in our view in the present moment. These objects could be specific people in the room or nearby objects. Next, we should zoom into four sounds we can hear. These sounds could be voices, the sound of tapping, or typing on a keyboard. Then, focus on three physical sensations in the body – perhaps the feeling of the back of a chair on your back, clothes against your skin, or the ground beneath your feet.

Next, focus on two scents. These could be the scent of perfume, incense, or flowers. Lastly, hone in on just one taste, which could simply be the natural taste that resides in your mouth. With each sense, narrowing down from five focal points to just one, we can mindfully transition from our sparse environment to within ourselves.

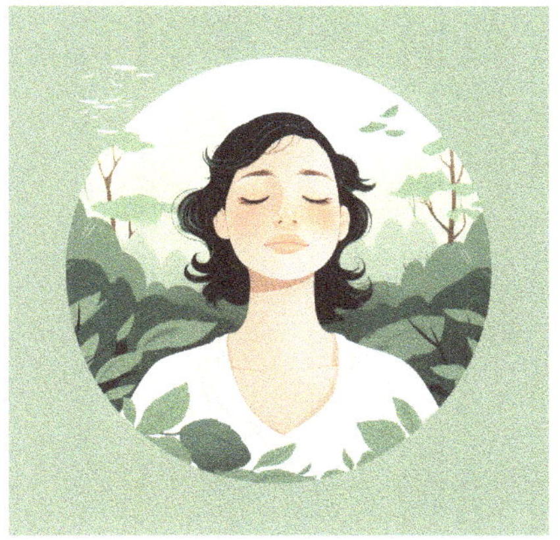

We can also see a sense of narrowing as we work through the senses. We are narrowing down from the sense that is most information-receiving (sight) to that which is the least information-receiving (taste). However, we can also see this visually: we have two eyes, two ears, two nostrils, and one mouth. We bring the senses down through the facial features to a single centred point at the mouth.

This strategy is a form of mindfulness, and can be practised on a regular basis in any space and at any time. To extend this mindful practice to help with pain or illness, we can visualise the concept of physically attaching our pain to the objects, sounds, sensations, feelings, smells, or tastes, on which we focus on. As we move through the layers from sight to taste, our pain or illness can be divided between a total of fifteen objects. This process allows us to transfer pain energy from within us to outside of us, and from our emotional inner selves to the physical world.

Sometimes, it is not as easy as it may seem to put this strategy into practice, especially since our surroundings are busy and our mind is easily distracted by worries of the past, present, and future. It is important to remain patient and encourage yourself to continue practicing. As always, we seek balance in Chinese medicine philosophy. Therefore, as this strategy works mostly to project feelings within to the outside world, we find balance by taking in our surroundings at the same time and allowing them to convert to feelings within us.

This outside-in healing mechanism is more useful when we are in a rather healthy state, and we are only seeking to improve our current health. One way of practising this, is through visualisation, often aided by closing the eyes. In this way, we close off one active sense (sight). Then, as we observe our surroundings through other senses, we can direct our remaining focus towards the feelings generated within us.

For self-reflection …

In which environments do you feel calm or at peace?

What are the specific aspects of these environments that bring you to a moment of calm?

How might you be able to look for these characteristics in environments in which you feel stressed?

WITHIN OUR ENVIRONMENT

Part 3

TIME AND SPACE

We all live busy lives, and often, when we are unwell, we find that making time to heal is difficult and disruptive. Clients also often note that a key trigger for stress is the thought that they are so busy, and that their schedules seem to be packed all the time.

When an individual is healthy, time remains a priority. Without the burden of pain or immediate need of healing, individuals have the luxury of organising their time for daily activities. However, when an individual is in the process of healing, time is not something that can be prioritised. Rather, space enables healing. It is impossible to know for sure how long it may take to heal completely. As a result, it can be impossible to plan out time in the way that we would usually hope to. Instead, it is important that we turn our attention to spatial awareness and our appreciation of it. The more we focus on where we are in space, the more effectively healing will progress.

This is a concept that we often see in mindfulness, a meditative practice during which individuals are encouraged to hone in on the sounds, smells, and sensations of their location, rather than where they are in time. This level of focus heightens our ability to think presently and thus allows for healing.

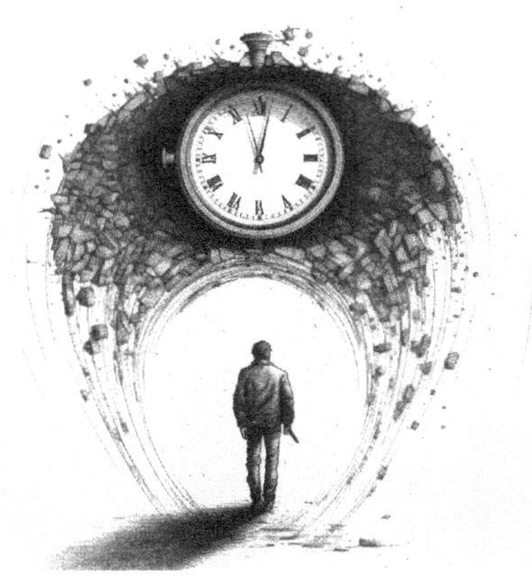

We can again see a connection with the universe, which has both spatial and time dimensions. Scientifically, all energy in the universe can be mapped onto a space-time diagram. This demonstrates how all objects, which are made of energy, can move both through time and space. Therefore, it is important not to neglect the value of space as well as time.

Many clients come into the clinic with a focus on how long it will take them to return to good health, or they ask for which specific dates and times they should return for follow-up treatments. Allowing the thought of time to become too overpowering can lead to a build-up of emotions and pressure in the mind due to forming expectations, which can disrupt the healing process. The build-up of emotions and pressure restricts the flow of healing qi.

We should take space into greater consideration when we are in the process of healing. By focusing on space, without a pressing urgency of time, we can more clearly see the situation at hand and find the most effective pathways for healing. One might say that time separates matter, drawing out stressful emotions, while space unites matter, as we can better visualise the bigger picture.

For self-reflection …

What are your busiest times of the year? How can you plan ahead for those times? Try to plan specific spaces that bring you peace and that you can immerse yourself within during these times.

THE UNIVERSE AND FLOW

Many clients are deeply immersed in their own health challenges and those of their loved ones. This focus is often a good thing, as we can focus on ourselves in a mindful and healing way. However, in these situations, we can sometimes forget that we are a part of a much larger and wide-reaching universe, and that connecting with the various external aspects of the universe can bring a different, yet still meaningful and mindful way of healing.

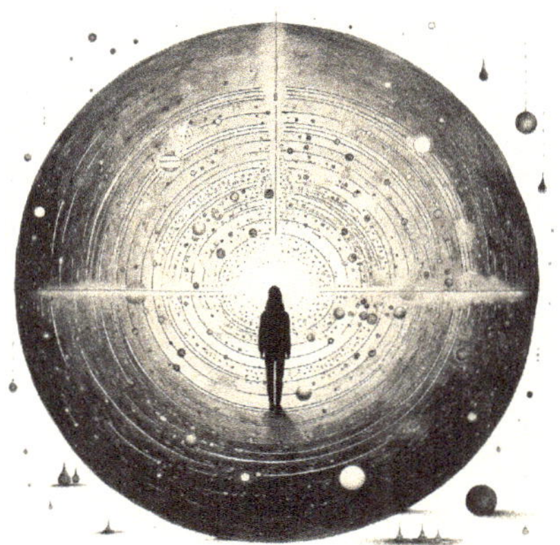

The universe is built around three aspects. We recognise them as information, materials, and energy. As humans, we rely majorly on our thoughts, consciousness, and perceptions to inform us on what is happening around us. We are incapable of comprehending the entire universe and will only ever have partial understanding, as goes with all the information we receive around us.

Additionally, the human mind is capable of processing feelings and individual thoughts and opinions. As a result, we will always have biased thoughts as it is difficult to draw our perceptions and views away from factual information.

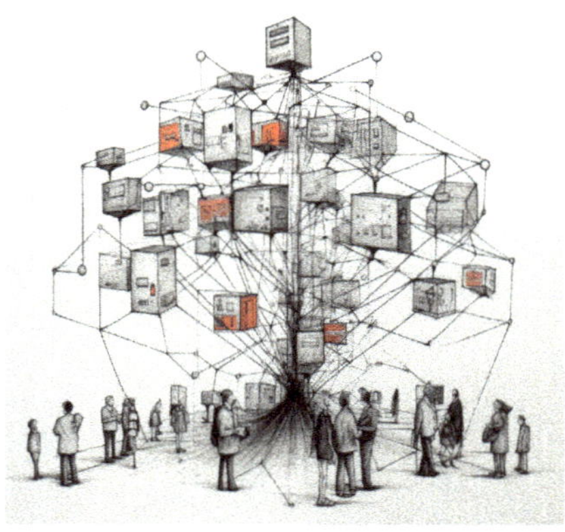

Different philosophers and therapists have different perspectives of the universe. This contributes to an abundance of information, based on each individual's identity and values. Therefore, it is not possible to know everything about our universe, and thus, the facts that exist in the universe will always be much greater than the thoughts we are capable of containing within our minds.

Matter and materials are responsible for the physical part of the world around us. Matter varies greatly – some matter is visible, like objects we hold in our hand or even our own bodies, while some matter is invisible, like the air and tiny molecules around us. Furthermore, all matter has a purpose, or a 'bias'. For

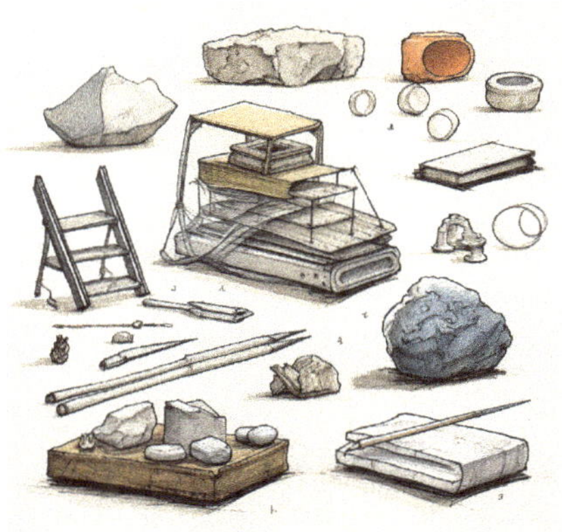

example, a t-shirt is made to be worn and a ball is made to be thrown. This same logic applies to human bodies. For instance, we learned to swim because we are capable of the skill, but we will never learn to fly without the assistance of other materials.

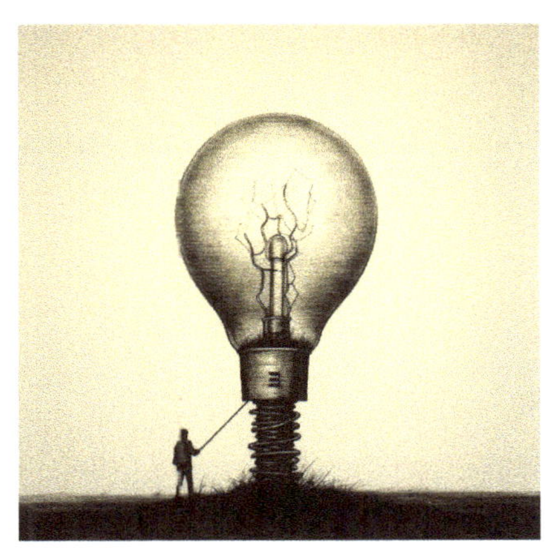

Unlike our thoughts and the purpose of matter, energy is unbiased. It exists everywhere in our universe in various forms. Energy is not limited to its uses or capabilities. It can be used to create, heal, and support, or to destroy, cause harm, or obliterate. Energy makes up everything, including matter, and therefore, we should make a conscious effort to connect with it. Traditional Chinese medicine specifically incorporates the flow of energy and balance into a patient's healing journey. This is a great way to directly connect the body, mind, and energy to establish mindfulness and nurturing care. When a person is mindfully and energetically connected to their body, they can more easily embrace their healing journey.

These three aspects, information, materials, and energy, also actively interact. For example, photos and art fall into the matter category. However, people connect with these pieces through emotion that is transmitted through different energy frequencies. Energy forms the means through which different aspects in the universe communicate. The more these aspects interact, the more energy is generated.

Energy and connection also manifest differently for every individual. This creates a range of frequencies of energy, which come together in harmony. Therefore, the more inter-action between forms, the greater harmony there is in the universe. In the context of healing, we gain external peace through medicine, but internal peace comes from connection with art and beauty, no matter how this manifests for each individual.

For self-reflection ...

When you appreciate art and beauty, do you connect mostly with the energy, materials, or the information that it repre-sents?

SCENT IN THE ENVIRONMENT

Noticing the scent in the environment may initially seem to be somewhat unrelated to our health and wellbeing. However, the ability to see how your energy relates to ordinary elements of the environment (such as scent) can create more far-reaching connections with the energy around you, not just within you.

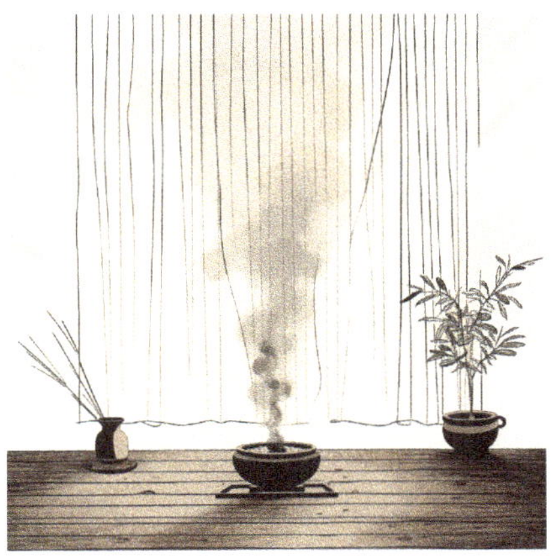

In traditional medicine, aroma has a major role when it comes to creating a safe, peaceful place, suitable for healing. When comparing incense to perfumes or room sprays, we should consider each person's individual taste and what is most balancing to one's wellbeing.

Incense often has a neutral scent that subtly fills the atmosphere around it. It is gentle and sets the tone of the environment, whilst still smelling pleasant and creating a peaceful setting. Incense is timeless - you do not need to change the scent often or worry about freshening the environment each day. Incense sets a long-term tone and intention for a space.

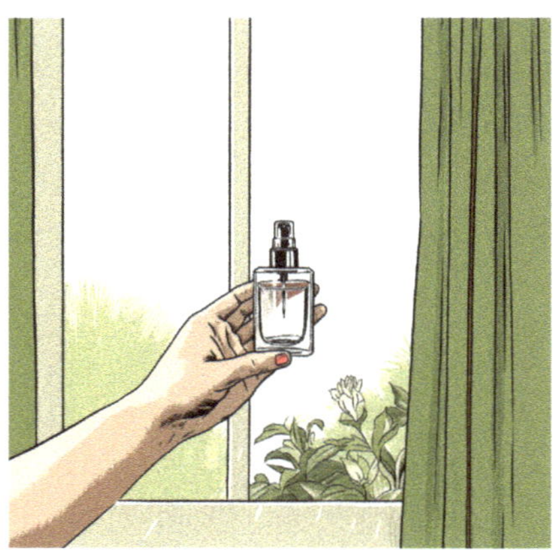

Perfume, on the other hand, can be overwhelming and overpowering and is usually associated with a personal taste - it is much less neutral. Perfume gives people a first impression of you as an individual. Whilst using a new perfume can be fun and exciting, it can easily be overused and long-term use can cause people to become obsessed, indecisive, or even depressed. In some cases, perfume can form a part of one's identity, and changing perfumes thus changes aspects of identity. To avoid becoming set in one way or developing an identity that is heavily influenced by scent, perfume should be changed or alternated regularly, and cleansed away at the end of each day.

The correct amount of perfume worn on a daily basis is subjective. However, too much perfume can cause physical illness, such as strong and long-lasting headaches. It is important to remember that the main purpose of a scent is to create a welcoming and peaceful atmosphere. Overusing perfume may also be perceived as covering up a part of ourselves or demonstrating too much intention to others. We show kindness and consideration for others and our environment by moderating our use of perfume.

While perfume introduces a much more sharp or defined scent, incense filters throughout a room with serenity and subtlety. Incense evokes greater humbleness, respect, and care, creating a field in which everyone in the space benefits from its effects.

Often, incense scents are quite neutral, and are therefore more inclusive to different tastes. As a result, incense scents feel much more welcoming than perfume scents. Sometimes, the scent of incense goes unnoticed as the scent blends into the atmosphere and heals in a hidden and concealed way. This may also be seen as a humbler quality of incense, which is not so typical of perfume.

For self-reflection ...

Are there certain scents that make you feel more relaxed or at peace?

Are there places in which you feel anxious? How might you be able to bring calming scents into these environments to create a more peaceful, healing atmosphere?

SUSTAINABLE HEALING

Part 4

SUSTAINABILITY

The word, 'sustainability', can have many different meanings. In the world today, we are urged to find ways of living more sustainably or protecting our environment more sustainably. These are examples of when the word 'sustainable' begins to create pressure. However, in order to solve pressing problems, we also need to see that we can heal sustainably and embrace the concept of being sustainable in a positive way. Sustainability does not need to cause stress or pressure, and we can work on developing this mindset even in small, unexpected ways.

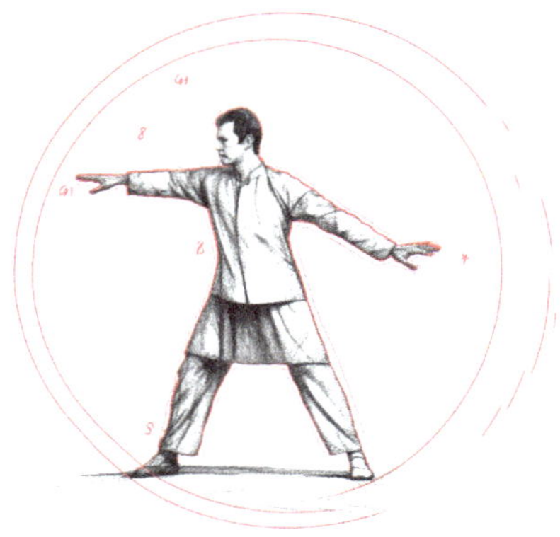

When an individual decides to embrace a journey of healing, they often attempt to dedicate themselves wholeheartedly to the process. However, for sustainable healing and growth, individuals should not embrace activities or healing with their full effort or exertion. Rather, they should use most of their effort in these activities, but reserve a portion of thought focused in the opposite 'direction'.

For example, in tai chi practice, physical movements or positions in a forward direction should be pushed forwards with most of our concentration. However, a small portion of our focus should remain pulling backward, in the opposite direction. In this context, one would pull their weight back into the back foot, while the forward foot steps and pushes forwards. This promotes greater balance and prevents us from toppling over.

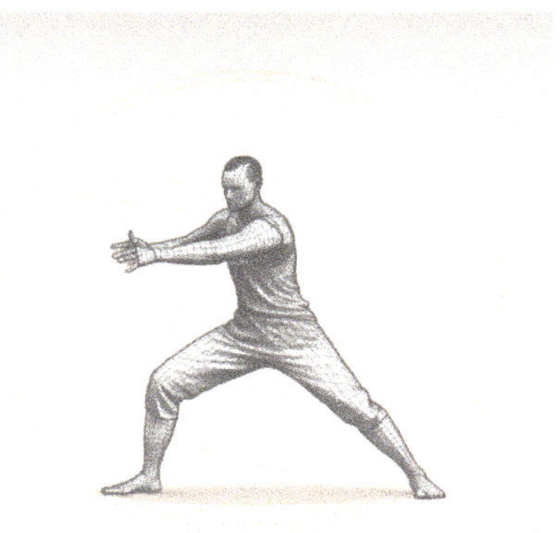

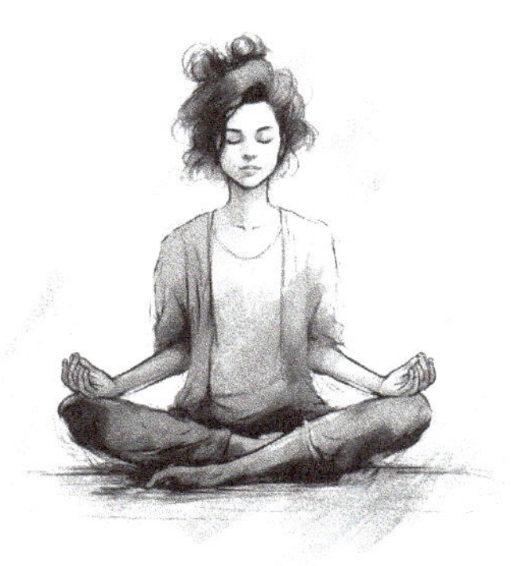

Another example is in mindfulness meditation. In mindfulness practice, an individual is often sitting still, which may make it seem as though it is possible to regulate the entire body at once. However, the reserved quality comes from our conscious effort to focus on specific parts of our body or surroundings. This focus on tiny aspects is a type of focus that also feels risk-free and sustainable. Using this small-focus strategy, we can protect our mind from becoming overwhelmed.

A physical example, is the well-known yin-yang logo. In the logo, we see the two curved shapes, where while one shape becomes thinner, the other shape becomes thicker and vice versa. This circular exchange allows for constant alternation between yin and yang, an exchange of both shape and energy. Thus, the exchange creates a sustainable flow.

In the earlier chapter, *Time and Space*, we explained that by alternating our focus between time and space, respectively depending on when we are in good health or when we are in need of healing, we are also creating sustainability.

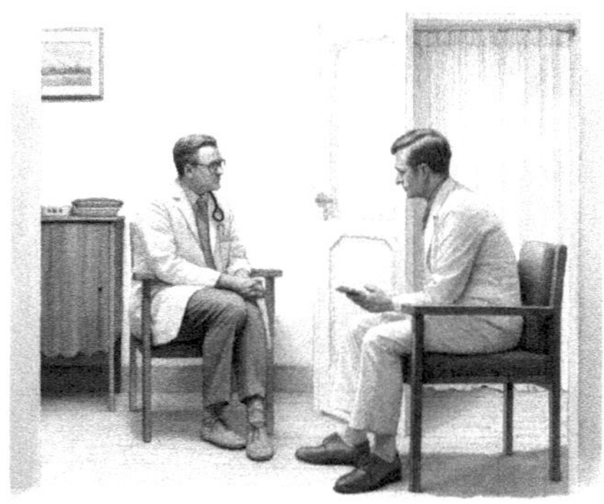

In the clinic, we also integrate sustainability into our healing plans. With clients, we remain transparent about where our plans are coming from, and how specific components of the plan play different roles in the healing process. This transparency enriches the collaborative relationship between the client and practitioner, and we can create a sustainable healing partnership.

For self-reflection ...

Can you recall any experiences in which you have felt quickly burned out? Do you feel that you may have put too much focus on one element of these experiences that may have caused this? How could you have held some opposite energy to have prevented this?

PRACTITIONER AND PATIENT

During an initial consultation with a new client, it is routine for the practitioner to give the patient an assessment. It is also important to recognise that this is the patient's opportunity to give the practitioner an assessment as well. This way, we can identify how the practitioner and patient can best work together throughout the healing journey. An analogy of poor alignment between a practitioner and a patient might be an ocean being held within a jar – this is a system in which the elements within the system do not support one another.

Healthy alignment between the practitioner and patient promotes the sharing of knowledge and experience. It is important that there is no sense of authority over one partner in the relationship, as this can lead to a one-sided energy imbalance, which does not support energy-based treatment in any way.

The practitioner and patient share equal roles and responsibilities in a recovery journey. Since Chinese medicine is based on energy flow, it is important that both the patient and therapist are aligned with the goal of removing energy

blocks and reach a level of understanding and trust throughout this process.

The patient plays a significant role in their own healing
journey, by being willing to receive treatment and embrace
changes to energy flow in their body. Maintaining a positive
attitude and taking care of themselves throughout the healing process, even when they are not being treated regularly,
will help to improve general wellness and the overall flow of
energy in the body.

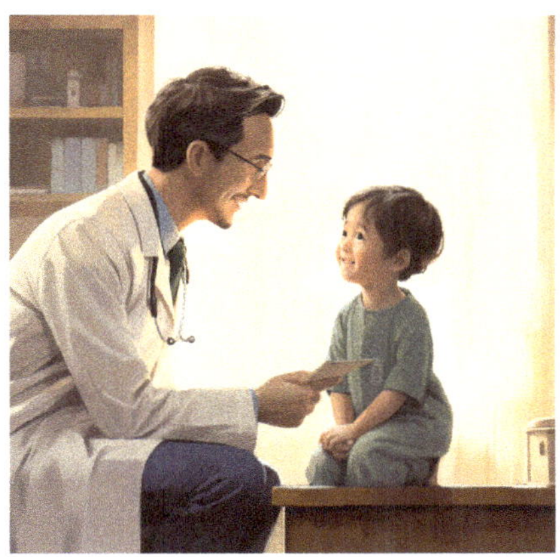

The practitioner should remain focused, determined, and
conscious of their posture and breathing while delivering
treatment. The practitioner delivers treatment with their
hands and can work to precisely distribute energy throughout the patient's body. Beneficial tools such as acupuncture
needles, cups, or herbal medicine are often used to assist and
amplify the effectiveness of healing.

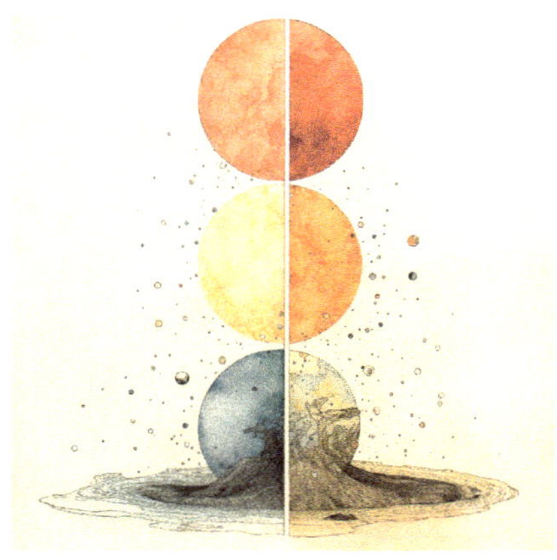

We can visualise the connection between the practitioner and the patient as the 'middle-layer' of three overall layers in our universe. The most expansive layer involves complex concepts, involving questions about the meaning of life or the role of humanity. The most narrowed or specific layer delves into our inner self and identity. Interactions between people or with the environment fall into the intermediate layer - this is where the practitioner-patient connection lies. It is within this middle layer that interactive energy is at its peak, exchanging rapidly between people, places, and objects. Therefore, we can see that the relationship between a practitioner and a patient should be active in communication, trust, and overall interaction.

For self-reflection ...

What do you and your practitioners have in common? What are your shared values and goals?

Are there ways in which you and your practitioners can communicate more effectively?

BALANCE OF THE ELEMENTS

The five elements are a basis of Chinese medicine philosophy. When clients want to learn more about this, the most important aspect to learn is that the five elements are not rigid or definitive concepts. Rather, the five elements represent different directions in which energy tends to flow. For example, a balance of the five elements implies that energy is flowing evenly in multiple directions. In this way, the balance of the elements correlates to an awareness of the space around you.

Chinese medicine's five elements are wood, fire, water, earth, and metal. Each element influences another element. One might visualise this as a five-point star, where each point symbolises a different element, and each element flows onto the next in a circular motion.

Issues can arise if there is imbalance between the elements. For example, if one element is too strong, other elements may be sedated and have less positive influence on the body. Conversely, if one element is too weak, there would be too much power and control given to other elements. In both scenarios, imbalances are emphasised and can grow into even greater imbalances.

We heal to mend imbalances; however, it is also important to take a non-full-on approach to maintain balance throughout the whole process. For instance, if an individual feels cold, instead of immediately turning to remedies solely representative of the fire element, we should take subtler steps of healing. This might involve remedies that include some characteristics of the fire element, but also some characteristics of the water element to prevent a major change to the person's elemental composition, and thus further imbalance. This conservative yet intentional approach to healing has been a central part of Chinese medicine since its beginnings in ancient times. The careful consideration of the amount of each element in the healing process, aiming to create balance both in the result of and during the process, may be considered an art in itself.

So far, we have mainly discussed the five elements simply in terms of their names: fire, earth, metal, wood, and water. However, we can also categorise many different concepts, functions, and special attributes into these five elements.

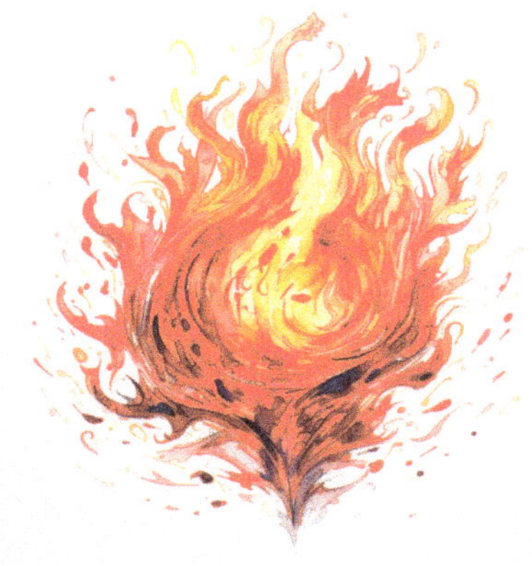

For example, with the fire element, we associate the colour red, the feeling of rigorousness, warmth, and enthusiasm. The category title, 'fire', is just a term that aids communication and understanding about the element.

Just as one element that is too strong will affect another element, we can now see that this effect applies to broader categories of concepts and objects, including emotions, body movements, and even beliefs. Let us analyse the case of the fire element having too much power, which we might see in the form of heat within the heart. This could be experienced as strong, overwhelming passion in the heart, or heaty, congested discomfort in the chest area. In this case, we could use healing methods that impose small amounts of fear or moreover the consciousness of the presence of fear, as fear is a concept associated with the water element. Alternatively, we could consider healing through our physical movements. For example, we should contrast fast, dynamic, fire-element movements with soft, gentle, water-element movements.

Overall, the key to achieving balance, is to apply character-istics of another element to reduce the power of a dominant element. Note that this concept is related to those detailed in the *Conceptual Spheres* chapter.

For self-reflection ...

What characteristics of your current treatment plan can you connect to the five elements? Could this give you a hint of which element(s) you are lacking more of?

LEVELS OF HEALING

Chinese medicine focuses on the concept of centralising energy. This relates to a conceptual 'middle'. The 'middle' has many interpretations. In a broader sense, the 'middle' might be the centre of the universe, or geographically, the 'middle' might be the Earth's equator. Both are examples of 'middles' that are assumed but not necessarily confirmed by factual evidence. The only centre we can truly depend on, is that which lies within ourselves. This is the centre that also relates to our healing journey.

The healing process involves all five senses. However, different treatment plans may target certain senses over others. Furthermore, each sense tends to have a different level of direct impact on a person's health, and we can rank these levels of impact from least to most directly impactful. The different 'levels of healing' are described as follows.

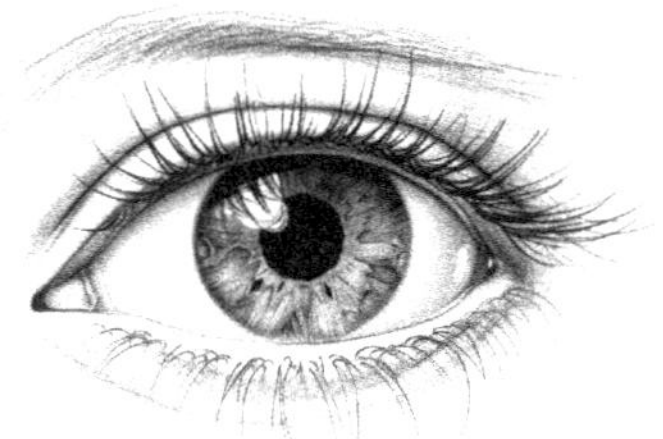

Lowest Level: Sight

Every individual has a different perspective of the same object or experience, resulting in each person being impacted differently by what they see. This is one of the reasons why sight has the lowest level of impact: we are simply affected differently by the things we see, and there is therefore a level of uncertainty associated with how sight will affect us. We can also consider that simply relying on symptoms that we can physically see to recognise illness or pain is only a surface level degree of self-analysis. We can often deduce much more about our wellbeing by involving our other senses.

Low Level: Smell

Scents also have a different effect on different individuals. For some, a certain smell may trigger old memories or induce instinctive feelings or emotions. Scent is also a component of how one presents themself to the world, through perfumes and cologne, or how one might welcome others into their home, through candles and incense. People naturally associate fond memories with

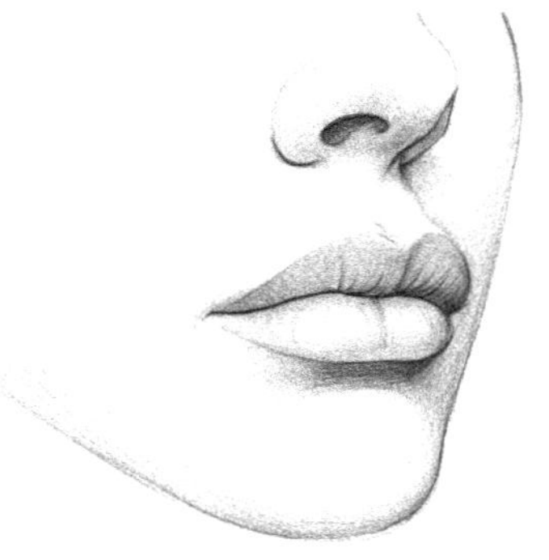

specific scents, and often, if we are met with the same aroma years later, those memories and feelings naturally resurface.

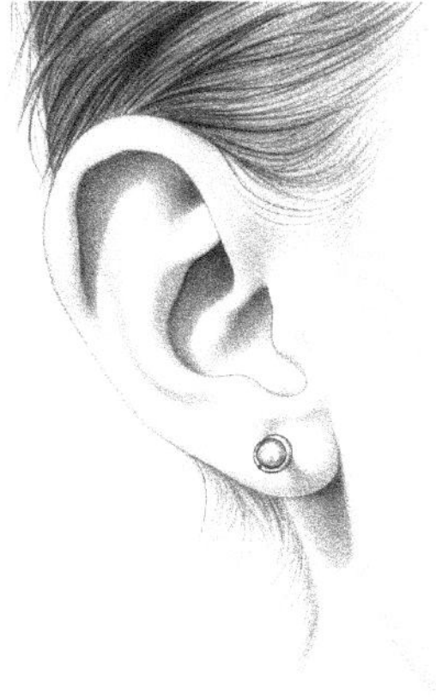

Medium Level: Sound

Our hearing is switched on constantly, and often, we cannot control what we hear – it happens subconsciously and without much effort. It is one of the primary ways in which we receive information from the world around us. However, hearing is not limited to voices and the sounds of moving objects in the environment. Sound is energy - a vibration. We can filter through different frequencies of sound vibrations, which allow us to hear pitch and interpret music. This can provoke emotional responses in humans, and, just like the Low Level, can trigger memories.

High Level: Taste

Taste can be triggered by many things - a strong aroma, physically ingesting food, or even simply imagining a meal. When we are deprived of food and nutrients, our emotional and physical state begins to deteriorate. As soon as we begin to fuel the body with the nutrition it needs, we tend to quickly start to experience improvement as the body has received new energy. Food is fuel and powers your body directly. Our nutrition in-take is also something over which we have some control – we decide what we put into our bodies.

Advanced Level: Touch

We usually have full control over how we use touch to treat ourselves and others, through remedial massage or acupuncture, for example. Therefore, touch is the sense which is most likely to produce highly meaningful and intentional health improvements.

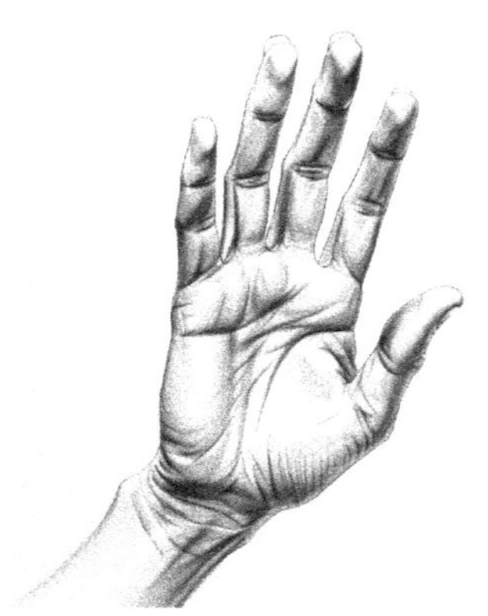

Regardless of whether a sense is ranked at a high or low level, all levels are powerful and practical in the healing process. It is important to remember that these rankings are based on the amount of healing one may experience following treatment that involves a particular sense over the other senses. However, there is not really a 'best' level. The greatest healing comes from a combined effort across various senses. Thus, it can be highly beneficial to create a healing environment that is accessible to all the senses.

Though there are many different functions associated with each level of the senses, the way we receive information should not always be based solely on this hierarchy of senses. For example, when clients are receiving treatment, they are often lying down in a position that is highly yin-dominant. Therefore, they are encouraged to only focus on the visualisation of their energy physically raising them upwards in this position, and thus involving more of a yang element. This single focus is simple, yet powerful, and allows the individual's clear focus to guide them towards recovery and healing. If, however, an individual was asked to imagine taking air in through the nose, into the lungs, and then connecting the sensations of exhaling with tension releasing through certain muscles in the body - there is now too much information. In this case, the individual's mind must leap between various different thoughts, complicating the focus on recovery. The longer the instruction is, the more distracting from the main purpose of treatment it can be. This somewhat relates to the concept that 'less is more'. Overall, we benefit more from simple information.

For self-reflection ...

When you are practising mindfulness, meditation, or tai chi, which sense do you feel that you can most naturally connect with? Notice what thoughts come to mind in response to that sense.

How can you focus on the other senses to bring more balance to your perception of the world?

TWO CYCLES OF FIVE ELEMENTS

Some clients already have a basic understanding, or have at least heard of the five elements in Chinese medicine philosophy prior to arriving at the clinic. However, this concept is much more intricate and interconnected beyond first glance. For those with an open mind and a desire to learn more about Chinese medicine, we like to introduce the two different cycles of the five elements and how these interact with us differently.

In Chinese medicine ideology, there are five main elements: wood, fire, earth, metal, and water. When we are healthy, this specific order of elements is most relevant. Each element generates the next element: wood generates fire, fire generates earth, earth generates metal, and so on. This is called a generation cycle, and is balanced across the five elements in a way that is repeating and circu-

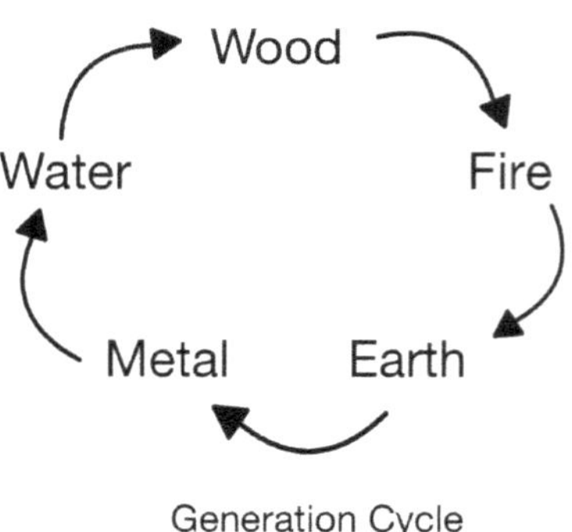

Generation Cycle

lar, when we are healthy. Balance and wellness are signified by a smooth and even flow of qi through the elements. As each element generates the next, qi is also generated, helping to regulate and enhance communication between the different elements.

On the other hand, when we are physically or mentally unwell, a different cycle reigns. This is known as a charged or controlling cycle. In this cycle, there is a new order of elements in play: water, fire, metal, wood, and earth. Each element controls or is 'in charge of' the next

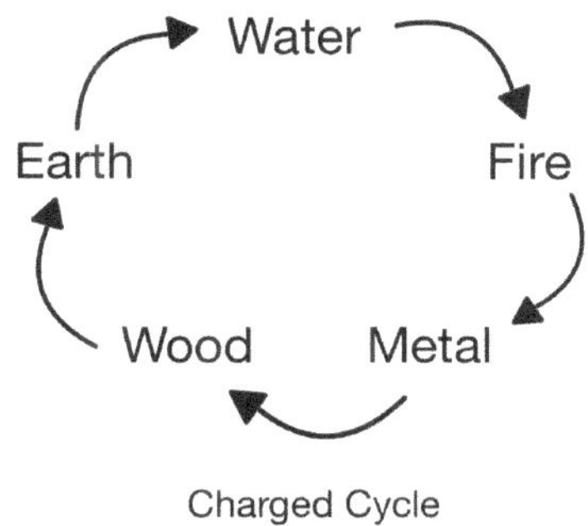

Charged Cycle

element. For example, water controls fire, fire controls metal, metal controls wood, wood controls earth, and finally, earth controls water. We can see that in this cycle, since each element both controls another element and is in control of another element, if one element becomes too strong (and thus controls another element with too much strength), an imbalance can arise. This imbalance disrupts the smooth and even flow of qi through the elements. The qi imbalance is what brings about the dominance of this charged cycle rather than the generating cycle, and with it, a specific healing force that works to neutralise the imbalance across the elements. Emotions can also be influenced by this charged cycle, and this is another complex yet significant application of this cycle.

Overall, the first cycle, which is the generating cycle, is nourishing and improves health and wellbeing when an individual is healthy. The second cycle, which is the charged cycle, works to correct imbalances of the elements and improves health and wellbeing when an individual is unhealthy.

For self-reflection …

Can you recognise if your past treatment plans may reflect one of the two cycles of five elements? When you are next feeling unwell, try to look for ways in which you can relate these cycles to your self-care or treatment plan.

ASPECTS INFLUENCING GENERAL HEALTH

Health professionals and practitioners usually give as much information as possible to their clients to ensure they are best equipped with information moving forward. At times, this can be overwhelming, and it can be useful to know some general ways of staying healthy.

Health, wellbeing, and happiness are influenced by multiple aspects, many of which are integrated and regularly influencing each other. In this chapter, we will cover a summarised list of ten major aspects that affect our general health.

First, calm and regulated breathing is important. Breathing should feel easy, in and out, allowing energy to transition from within us to our environment and vice versa. This process should be natural, without requiring much conscious thought.

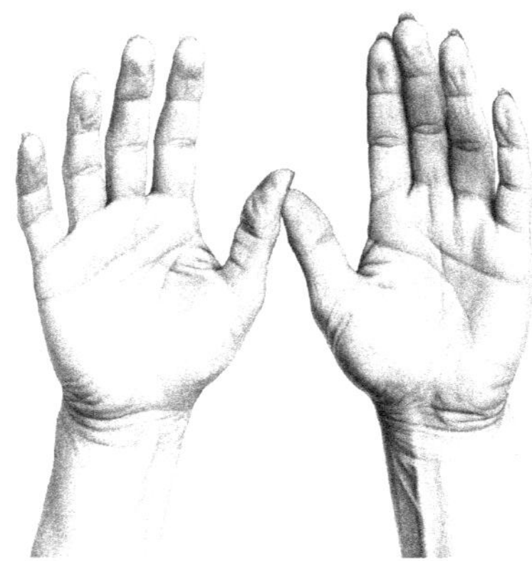

Second, we should be able to regulate sensations in our hands and feet, noticing whether they feel hot or cold, or are in pain, for example. Our hands and feet drive our sense of direction and initiative.

Third, our mind and eyes should be relaxed, but inter-linked, allowing us to look internally into ourselves as well as outwards. This means we can more mindfully connect with our internal thoughts and visualisations. We may visualise places of peace and healing when we practice mindfulness, or physical representations of emotions that we feel.

Fourth, our overall body should be relaxed, without strain, to allow for flexibility in our movements and a balanced flow of qi.

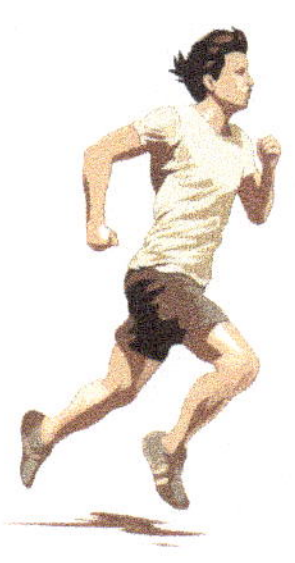

Fifth, physical movements should be smooth and natural. Beautiful movements come from a place of kindness, patience, and balance, and not from a place of tension.

Sixth. Our reactions to certain experiences should be without major tension, full-force power, or rigidity. This maintains our circular and elegant movements, and again encourages a healthy flow of qi.

Seventh, remaining in touch with our spirit is key. We should listen to our gut feeling and sense of spirituality when it comes to maintaining health.

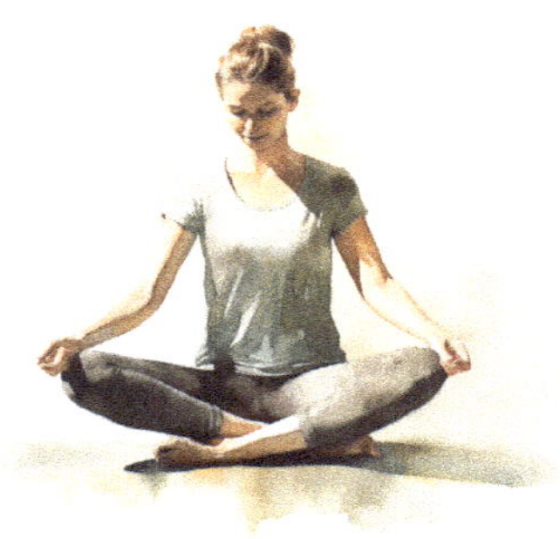

Eighth, our thoughts should be intentional, colourful, and varied, rather than dispersed and in-cohesive. This encourages healthy decision-making and balance.

Ninth, our communication and expression should be sincere, natural, and delicate. We should have intention in our expression, and should not feel rushed or pressured to express ourselves in a specific way.

Tenth, we should pay attention to our body posture. With a relaxed and non-sluggish deportment, we can invite qi to move calmly yet empoweringly around the body.

Knowing about these ten aspects will have a positive impact on a healing process. However, it is also important to know how to approach the healing process. This process can be summarised in five main steps.

The first step is all about gathering information. We should research and find out as much relevant information as possible about the situation at hand.

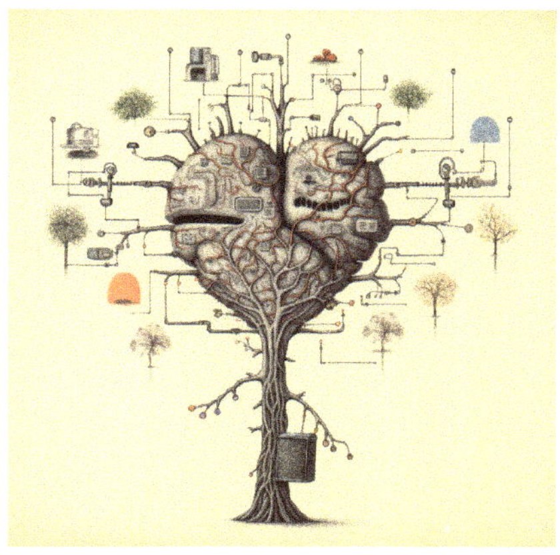

The second step involves planning. Now that we know what our situation entails, we need a plan of action and a commitment to the process. Often, healing is an ongoing process that requires consistent effort and motivation.

The third step is the actual implementation of the healing plan from the second category. It is important to remain focused on the plan, but still maintain an open mind should something cause the plan to unexpectedly change.

The fourth step involves reviewing the entire process - this step technically starts at the same time as the first step. It is valuable to take note of both the high and low points throughout the process to improve our approach to healing in future. This is where we reflect on where we are at the end of the process. What has changed? What should be done next? It can be difficult, but extremely powerful to be honest with oneself during this reflection period.

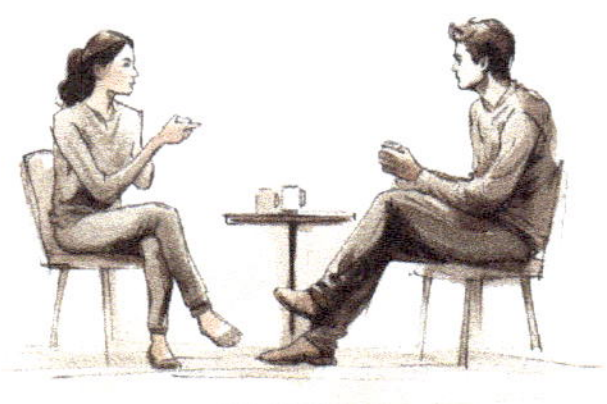

The fifth and final step is about sharing and reflecting to others how we have grown or changed as an individual. This is an outward version of reflection, that includes others in our progress and may encourage others to engage in similar growth.

For self-reflection ...

Which general aspects do you already regulate quite well?

Which general aspects can you focus on more? How will you do this?

ENERGY

Part 5

TYPES OF PAIN

Before we can begin to heal, we should spend time understanding the type and location of pain we are experiencing. Most individuals focus on the pain that they can physically feel when describing their symptoms. This is the most well-known type of pain, called 'expressive' pain.

Expressive pain, also known as 'yang' pain, involves feelings of soreness, aching, or sharp pains that we feel through obvious physical sensations. This pain comes from within us and expresses itself outwards into our consciousness. Though it is not always pleasant, expressive pain can be considered a good type of pain, because our body is readily alerting us of painful areas and we are usually able to take action to heal.

There is another, less well-known type of pain: hidden pain. Also known as 'yin' pain, hidden pain is not readily visible and does not present itself through obvious physical sensations or soreness. Rather, we can only know that hidden pain exists if we find it before we feel it. For example, during a massage therapy session, a massage therapist might locate a point of pain on the body that hurts to the touch, but was not evident prior to the massage session. We first locate this pain from outside our body and then feel it within our body.

Hidden pain can often be more concerning than expressive pain simply as it is not so easily visible.

Generally, in Chinese medicine, experiencing pain is the result of having energy blockages. The locations of energy blockages indicate where in the body there is too much accumulated energy. The meridians in the affected areas are thus full of energy that is not flowing to other parts of the body.

For more effective, harmonious healing, it is important to find and locate both types of pain, expressive and hidden, to implement healing strategies effectively. We should not solely focus on the expressive pain we feel, or express blame towards one part of the body that is causing the pain. Instead, it can be highly effective to seek out hidden pain that may be the underlying cause of expressive pain. By approaching from this deeper level of pain, we may find a way to mend the foundation of the more surface-level expressive pain, and remove all the pain completely.

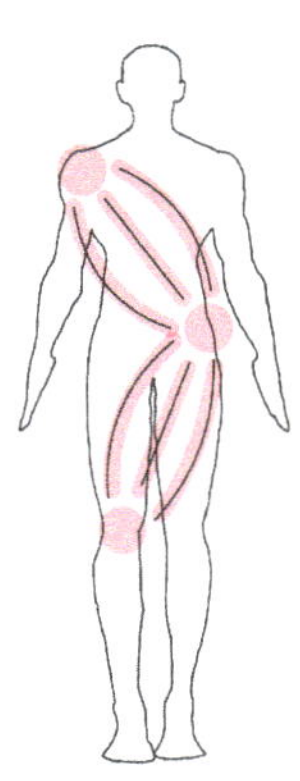

We often find it very effective to treat areas of the body that are distantly linked via meridians. These connective meridians are between the areas in which an individual may experience expressive pain, and areas in which we have found hidden pain. As well as being able to reveal more areas of hidden pain that may be contributing to expressive pain, we are able to cover a greater range of the body through the meridian network.

The energy build-up in affected areas of expressive pain can spread out, transform, or undergo a combination of both dispersal and transformation across the meridians. This energy will gradually reach the area being treated, thinning out the build-up and promoting a healthy flow of qi. In general, the process starts with the location of expressive pain, then the accumulated energy spreads across a larger area, and this process of energy-spreading repeats with different meridians, until no more build-up is evident.

For self-reflection ...

What are some examples of expressive pain that you regularly experience? Try to release your focus on these areas to allow for areas of hidden pain to come to light.

Next time you have acupuncture or remedial massage treatment, notice where the focus of the treatment is on your body. How might this relate to areas of expressive and hidden pain?

OPENNESS, CLOSEDNESS, AND TRANSITION

Most people have heard of the terms 'openness' and 'closedness' in the context of the mind. For example, when we feel that the mind is open, we may feel more positive towards new experiences, and when we feel that the mind is closed, we may feel more shut away from society. We can extend these states to our physical motions as well. On a regular basis, we naturally alternate between physical states of openness, closedness, and transition.

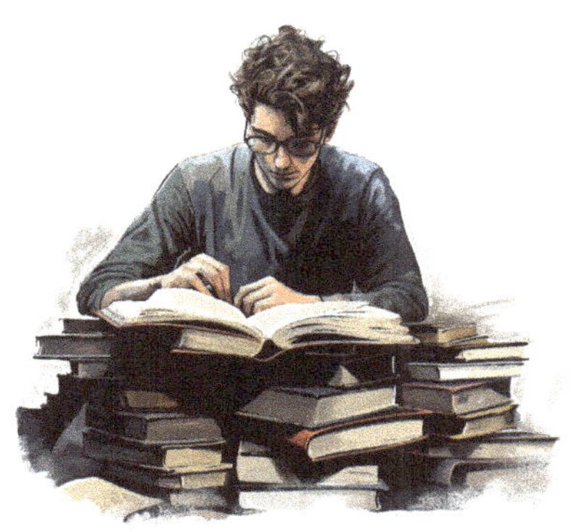

A state of openness may appear as body movements that stretch or expand into a bigger space with a sense of positivity. We might associate this idea with the concept of smoothness.

In contrast, a state of closedness might evoke feelings of withdrawal or conservation. Positive closedness can allow for internal peace and internal growth, and may be visualised as the gathering of body parts. Negative closedness can be associated with body movements that are rigid or flexed.

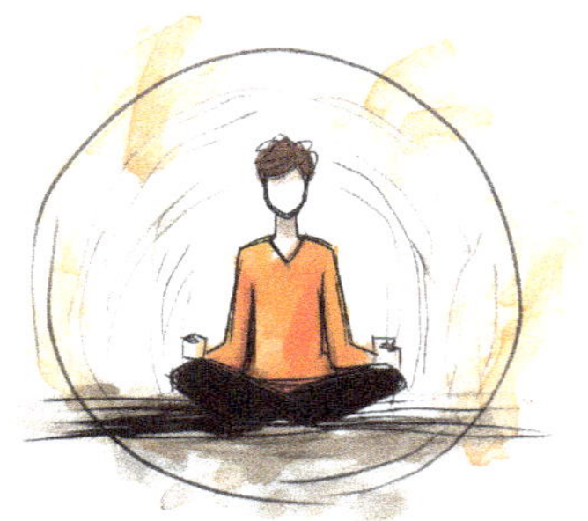

A state of transition is one that lies between states of openness and closedness. The transitional state encompasses movements that alternate between expanding and contracting physical movements, or movements that are unclassifiable between these categories.

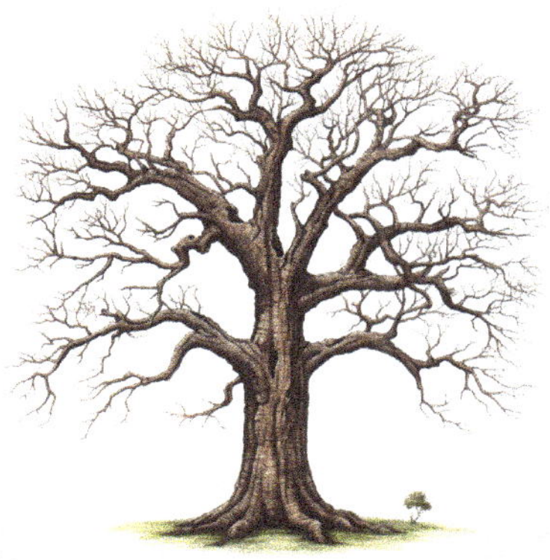

Meridians in our body also connect with our openness and closedness. Each meridian accesses energy and nutrition, and can shape our openness and closedness. Different meridians have different purposes, much like a tree: some meridians produce the flowers, some produce the leaves, and others strengthen the bark. Meridians allocate and distribute energy to different parts of the body, and also influence different characteristics seen in the corresponding areas of the body.

We can also analyse the states of openness, closedness, and transition in terms of our mind-body connection. Our body movements match our thoughts, and thus, our body's open, closed, and transitional states match our mind's respective open, closed, and transitional thoughts. When our body is in a closed state, we allow our mind to reflect internally, which allows for self-improvement and growth. When our body is in an open state, we allow our mind to embrace new knowledge and learn. When our body is in a transitional state, our mind can negotiate, contemplate, and debate prior to making decisions.

In this sense, our mind and body act as partners, much like the highly interactive relationship between yin and yang. By syncing these partners in a shared state of openness, closedness, or transition, we create an atmosphere of harmony, which is necessary for effective healing. Put simply, we should not only think about how we can best go about healing, but strive to unify the mind and body.

For self-reflection ...

Do you feel more naturally in an open, closed, or transitional state?

What physical activities or exercises could you do to access all three of these physical states?

PERCEPTION OF ENERGY

As individuals, we perceive thoughts and ideas in different ways. In the same way, we can perceive the concept of energy differently. This is something we often focus on when we meet new patients – broadening the mind to welcome new ways of thinking about energy and how it interacts with matter. This can help to create stronger connection between the patient and their healing journey.

Energy presents itself in many forms. We may be more familiar with perceiving energy as light or warmth, but energy can also come from pressure, expansion, or any change in an object's motion. For this reason, energy is not 'linear'. In other words, energy cannot be represented by a line or a two-dimensional sense of understanding.

There are several forms of 'energy medicine', including tai chi, cupping, and techniques that involve nature. Just as energy cannot be defined linearly, neither should methods of energy medicine treatment. One should not focus on one type of treatment to heal one specific issue as one remedy may not always help the same symptom.

Ideally, patients should focus on the sensations of energy they feel, using breathing techniques to do this. When we breathe, energy flows in and out. Therefore, breathing techniques allow us to visualise and connect with this alternating motion of energy in and out of the body.

We can also see that energy presents itself in the form of six main senses - in addition to the five traditional senses, we also count the mind's activity as a sense. These six senses correspond to six main body parts: the eyes (sight), nose (smell), ears (sound), tongue (taste), skin (touch), and brain (thought).

There is a connection here with the concept of the 'six roots' in Buddhist belief. These roots may be interpreted as channels of energy. In general, a channel is a space that allows for a substance (such as wind, water, or energy) to flow in a certain direction. The six associated organs each act as a channel of energy, allowing smell, sound, sight, and the other senses to flow in and out of us in the form of energy. As the senses flow, it can become very easy to begin associating strong feelings or preference towards certain sensations.

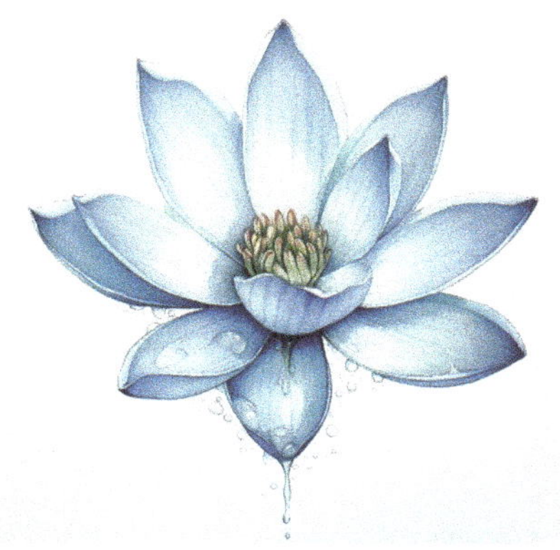

For example, a sweet-smelling flower would likely be identified as pleasant, while the feeling of a rough rock might introduce some inner stress or fear. However, energy itself cannot be strictly 'good' or 'bad' - it simply exists and transitions between different forms. In energy medicine, it is important not to allow ourselves to attach certain feelings to certain forms of energy.

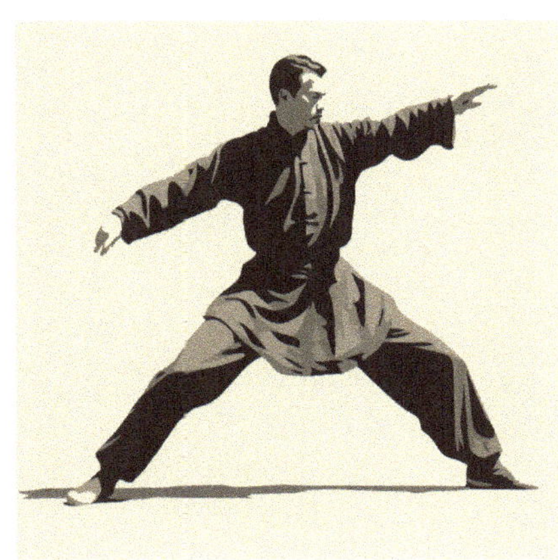

In tai chi, it is common to work towards maintaining calmness and serenity, bringing ourselves into a neutral state. This reduces the likelihood of attaching certain feelings and emotions to different sensations, keeping energy pure. When practising tai chi, try to keep your eyes half-closed and listen to sounds within your body. These are just two examples of ways we can achieve a neutral state amidst pure, cleansing, and healing energy.

For self-reflection ...

What image comes to mind when you think about the concept of energy?

Take notice of certain emotions you experience. How do your energy levels vary with these emotions?

LITERATURE AND ENERGY

Continuing from the last chapter about our perception of energy, one way of perceiving energy is through our own words and phrases. It is sometimes a surprise to people who have not heard of this representation of energy before – how can language carry energy?

Different types of words correlate with different energy levels and actions. Nouns (people, places, or things) carry weight and represent objects or concepts that are substantial and energy-holding. Verbs (action words) are very energetic, full of motion and movement. Adjectives (descriptive words) project passion, emotion, and human connection. Pronouns (eg. 'I', 'she', 'they', 'we') indicate a direction towards a person, place, or object. In other words, they indicate directions in which energy should be projected. Prepositions (eg. 'on', 'at', 'under', 'near') connect with spatial awareness, depending on comparative descriptions of locations. Words that describe degrees or quantities, such as 'very much' or 'a lot', are subjective and draw energy to one area more than another. Conjunctions (eg. 'and', 'furthermore', 'but') bring more logic and dimension into our meaning, as we are able to associate and connect concepts with different situations.

Language, therefore, has a physical representation related to their different actions, purposes, and energy levels. This means that if we repeat our style of speaking by using the same type of words, sentence structures, grammar, and tone, we are prone to accumulating too much of the same type of energy. We should also consider that changing our speaking style is important to balance our constantly changing body, environment, and thoughts. Information is energy, and one should therefore aim to maintain balance through variation. In meditation, it is common practice to make the sound 'ommm'. This sound does not carry any single direction or resemble a certain type of word. Instead, it is a pure, cleansing sound that reaches over the range of an area. This purifying sound creates balance, and similar sounds are used in sound therapy.

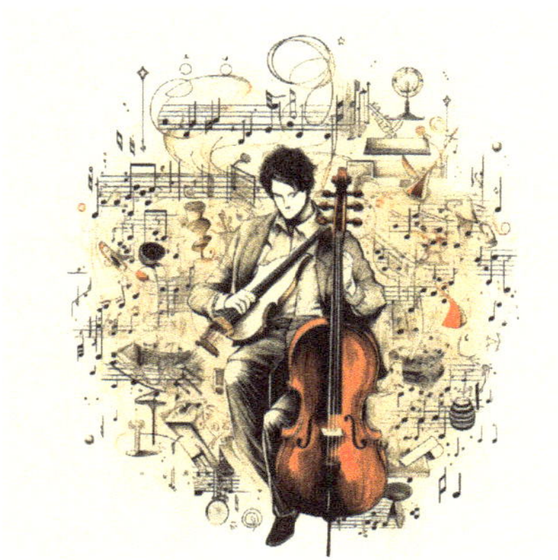

Some forms of music, however, are very rule-based, such as classical music. The classical music structure is quite repetitive and strict, and may create imbalances. Therefore, it is important to remember to vary the type of music we listen to.

Understanding the way that different words and language carry energy can be very powerful. With this knowledge, we can communicate in a meaningful and effective manner. After all, language is the main way in which we present our thoughts, emotions, and beliefs, and is a way of influencing ourselves, others, and the world.

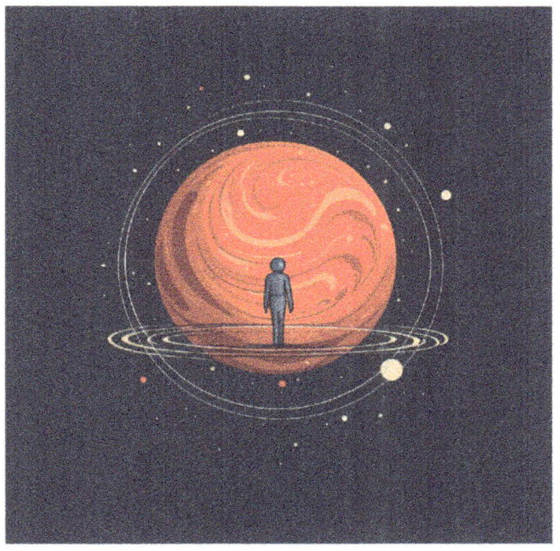

If we analogise our body as a mini-universe, our words take meaning and information, and are projected as energy, perhaps taking the form of planets orbiting around us. In other words, our words, which carry energy, are a solar system around us. They contribute to our system of energy - our words directly affect us. As a main principle, we should pay attention to the structure and variation of our words, expressions, and meanings, and be conscious of how we send messages into the world.

For self-reflection ...

Try to examine your style of communication (most find it easiest to see this in their writing style). Are there certain patterns in your language use? Challenge yourself to articulate your thoughts and ideas with different words and sentence structures.

YIN AND YANG IN BODY POSITIONS

The terms 'yin' and 'yang' are likely the most well-known in Chinese medicine. Most clients have heard of these terms before seeking out Chinese medicine treatment. However, these two concepts are quite intricate and interconnected, and knowing more about yin and yang often brings a new sense of understanding of Chinese medicine treatment, and health and wellbeing in general.

Yin is energy that is associated with coldness, femininity, night-time, rest, and horizontal shapes. Conversely, yang is energy that is associated with warmth, masculinity, day-time, activity, and vertical shapes. We can also see combinations of yin and yang in different structures and body positions.

In a typical standing position, an individual usually occupies a vertical, yang position. While sitting in a chair, our back and lower legs are vertical and our upper legs are horizontal, creating a combination of yin and yang.

Even though balance is often a good thing and is regularly sought out in Chinese medicine, the mixture of yin and yang in the seated position means it is a position that is very comfortable and easy to remain in for large amounts of time. In comparison, standing up, which is a yang position cannot be sustained for too long. The most dangerous aspect of the seated position, however, is the way in which yang (in the vertical, upright back) is always in the top part of the position (above the horizontal lap). This can create too much separation between the yin and yang energies, leading to an imbalance. We might visualise this effect as a helium-filled balloon, where no matter how many times you push the balloon downward, it will always float back up. This can become dangerous as we are not varying our position or allowing energy to change and transition – it is sometimes said that the seated position is the closest to death for this reason.

Walking or running positions are upright and vertical, but also moving forward. Therefore, this position is double yang (visualise a vertical line that is also moving forward through space). Rolling on the floor occupies a horizontal position, which would suggest the presence of yin energy. However, due to the rolling motion, there is also a vertical component and hence yang in the position too.

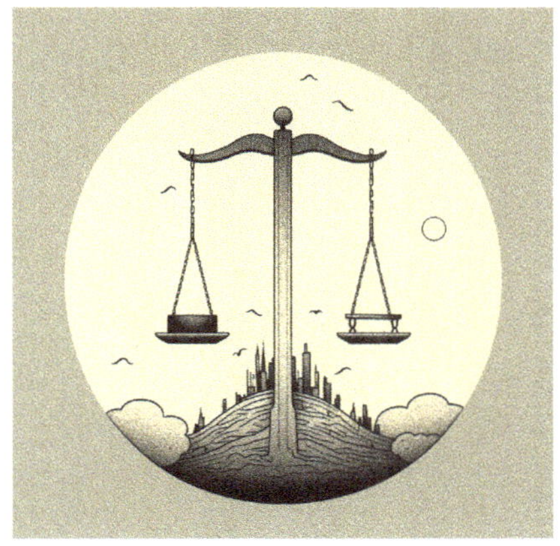

Overall, Chinese medicine values neutrality, balance, and harmony between yin and yang. Thus, we should remain active and in a state of constantly changing positions. There are currently five main body postures that we commonly see in society: standing up, lying down, walking, sitting, and crawling. It can be said that in the past, all these common positions were balanced, as individuals would generally occupy each position for roughly the same amount of time throughout their lifetime. Only recently, sitting has become much more prominent over the rest of the positions, creating an imbalance.

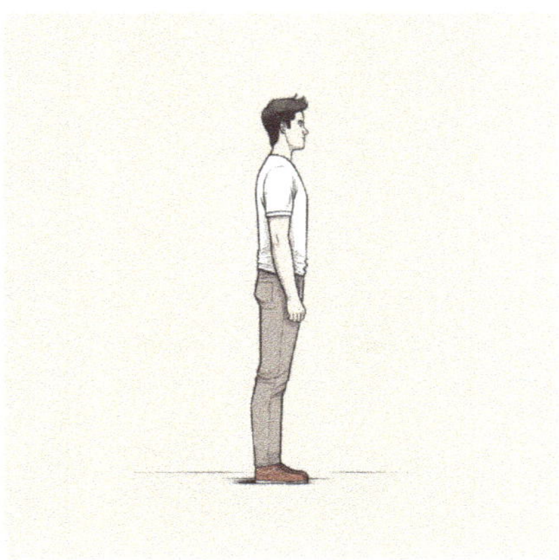

The standing position (yang) feeds our curiosity. It is a very motivated position, allowing us to investigate and encouraging us to make important decisions in life. The lying down position (yin) allows us to take rest and heal. The walking position (double yang) activates our survival instincts, including fight or flight reflexes. We can escape from danger, physically move to different places, and accomplish tasks to stay alive.

In the last five or six centuries, the sitting position has become one of the most common positions in civilisation, and a natural part of our daily lives. However, we may interpret this position as man- made. This is because it is not a position that guarantees our ability to survive - we stand to make life-changing decisions, we lie down to recover and regain energy, and we walk to achieve basic survival tasks - but we do not necessarily need to sit down. Some may argue that the sitting position is the position in which we can consume food at a meal, for example. Though it may be the social norm to have meals while seated, it is not necessary for survival. Rather, seated meals are a luxury and a choice.

As explained earlier, the seated position occupies both yin and yang qualities in the way that there are both vertical and horizontal components in the position. Hence, the seated position spans a wide range of energy across both dimensions, and yet, it is confined to the limiting structured shape of a chair. In the earlier chapter, *Visibility of Emotions* (in Part 2 of this book), we discussed how structured, distinct shapes can hold a lot of energy. Though we may be achieving a sense of balance from the presence of both yin and yang in the seated position, we simultaneously impose an imbalance as we essentially aim to squeeze a large amount of energy into a structured shape.

Therefore, the crawling position should be adopted more to balance the instability of the seated position. It is true that crawling is common for young children who are learning to walk, and we can see that during this time, young children are much like sponges, able to learn and grow at a rapid pace, and adapt quickly in new situations. After we learn to walk and through adulthood, crawling becomes absent. The crawling position may be interpreted as the opposite to sitting. Like the sitting position, the crawling position also involves both yin and yang across both vertical and horizontal components. However, the crawling position is not limited to a distinct structure and there is more space for the combination of yin and yang energy to disperse. As a result, we can see that the crawling position balances the imbalances from the structured sitting position.

There is a correlation between our body positions and our abundance of yin and yang energies, which directly affect our health and wellbeing. If we are unwell, we usually need more yin and thus tend to lie down and rest (the horizontal position). When we have been lying down too much, and thus accumulating too much yin, we should stand up and walk around more to invite more yang into our energy system. We should also be varying our positions: sitting, crawling, rolling, jumping, and more. Varying our body positions helps us maintain balance between yin and yang.

For self-reflection …

Approximately how many hours in a day do you spend sitting down?

Are there daily activities you perform seated that you could replace with a standing position?

LANGUAGE, COMMUNICATION, AND UNDERSTANDING

We may not always be aware of it and the concept may seem confusing at first, but our thoughts can never truly be complete. In other words, our thoughts can never be a perfect representation of the vast concept of truth. Furthermore, the truth always has some degree of uncertainty related to it, and even the parts of the truth that we may understand cannot be perfectly expressed in our internal thoughts. The limit of our expression continues when we attempt to use language to express our understanding to others. Our vocabulary is simply not extensive enough to perfectly match our thoughts and the truth beyond that.

As discussed in the chapter, *Literature and Energy* (Part 5), different types of words carry different levels of energy. Since we are already limited by language in our expression, it is important to vary our use of language to promote positive energy flow within ourselves, and between us and the outside world. When trying to convey meaning, individuals should not simply repeat sentences, speed up or slow down their talking pace, or raise or lower their volume. These adjustments do not alter the types of words used and are therefore considered one-dimensional changes. For more effective meaning and thus greater positive energy, individuals should always vary their communication styles.

A similar concept relates to the concept of asking 'good questions' and receiving 'good answers'. For example, if an individual is not finding the answer they are looking for, rather than asking the same questions and searching for different answers, they should focus on asking new questions. This method changes the path of research significantly and is much more likely to reveal new answers and knowledge.

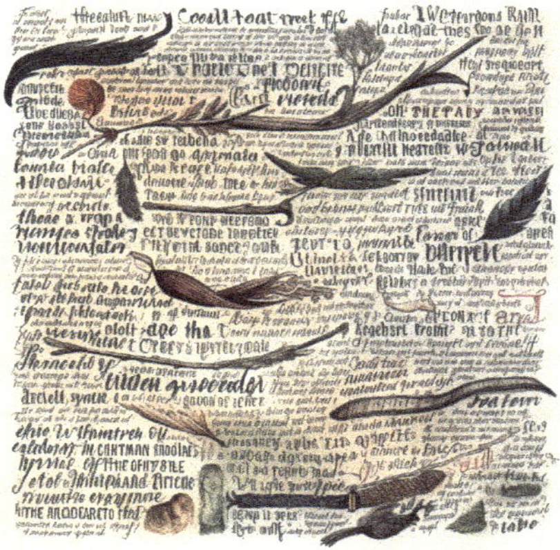

Therefore, we should be varying our vocabulary and sentence structure not only to balance the types of energy we carry and project, but also to ask more meaningful, varied questions. The concept of varying the way we communicate may seem daunting, especially as there are already well-defined rules in society regarding grammar and use of tenses. Even though there is a recommended or a specified 'best' way of communication, it is important to challenge ourselves to find variations in our spoken language. Correct grammar and use of tenses are still important, but variation is what promotes a healthier being. We should aim to find a balance between correct grammar and varied language.

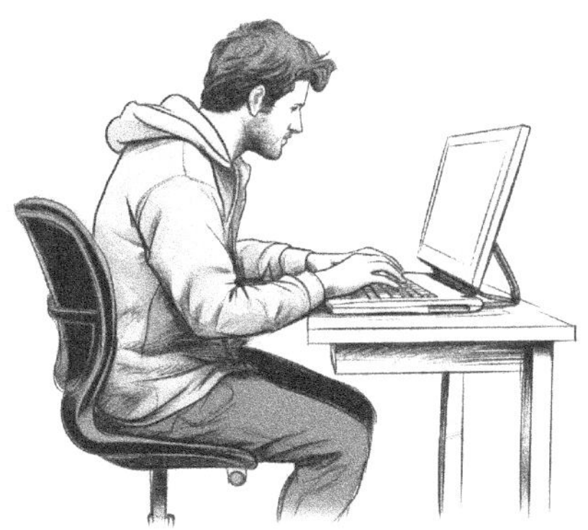

As an example, we can look to artificial intelligence (AI) platforms on the internet. We find that by asking AI questions in different ways (with different expression styles and sentence variation), AI will return a range of answers. Similarly, AI may return the answers with the same meaning, but in different structures or words. This means that AI can express meaning in many different ways, and can thus communicate with more people, and expand its own knowledge.

Repeatedly using similar types of language, words, or expression style, or looking for the same answer without changing the questions asked can lead to energy blockages. Certain forms of energy will overload (from repeated words) and draw from other forms of energy (from underused words). This challenge may manifest in health issues or negative effects on our wellbeing.

For self-reflection ...

When you are trying to find the answer to a specific question, think about the ways in which you can rephrase the question to have the same meaning.

Are there synonyms you can use for certain words?

Are there metaphors that can help you visualise your questions better?

BALANCING QI AND BLOOD CIRCULATION

Throughout these chapters, it is evident that the five senses hold great importance in our wellbeing. All these five senses are controlled from areas in the face and head: in the eyes, ears, nose, mouth, and skin. Because of this, it can be easy to attribute a lot of our energy and focus to this area of the body.

Wherever we draw our focus to, is where qi is directed. Additionally, where intention and qi are directed, there is also a concentration of blood. Blood will tend to circulate in the areas where qi is prominent, and can cause congestion in these areas.

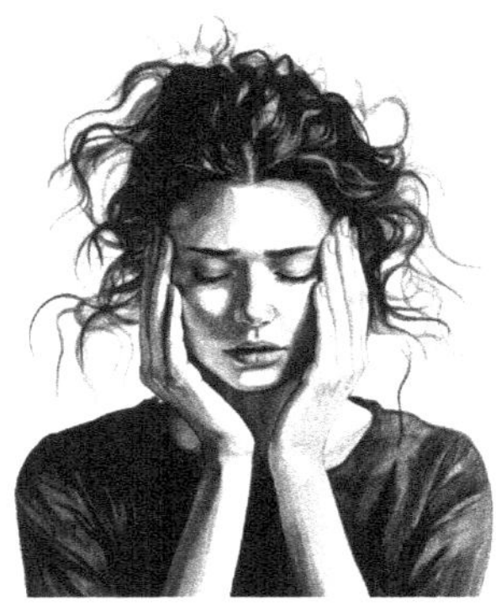

For example, someone who is highly stressed most of the time, might draw too much qi and blood to the front part of their head, causing heaviness in the head, and a metaphorical feeling of falling downward due to the weight. The individual may experience headaches and pain in this frontal area of the head. This concept of qi and blood circulation originates from concepts in tai chi practice. Tai chi is not just about slow and steady movements, but also visualisation within the mind, specifically of gentle changes in the body.

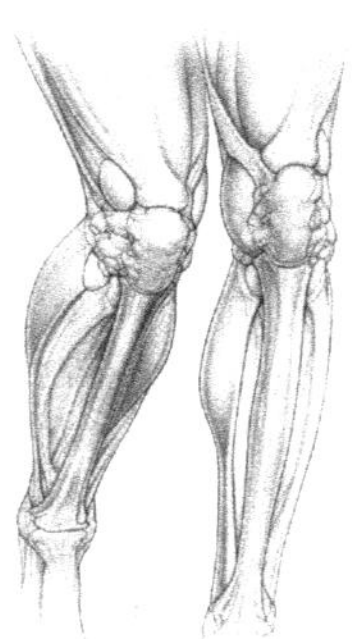

There are two ways of using visualisation to regulate the body and circulation. We can first use visualisation to prevent injury or pain. For example, if you bend one knee, you may notice the mind's focus shift to the bent knee area. Therefore, qi flows there to support the knee, and as a result, blood circulates there too. This helps to maintain a healthy blood and qi flow, and strengthens the knee against future injury or pain while it is in a vulnerable, bent position.

We can also use visualisation to release pain sensations. We should recall that tension is a feeling that comes from energy build-ups and blockages in qi meridians. Therefore, the goal is to guide energy away from the blockage to allow it to spread evenly throughout the body and gradually remove the blockage. In this scenario, focus on where the tension is and visualise a different area on the opposite side of the body. For example, if there is tension in the left shoulder, the right hip is somewhat opposite the left shoulder, and this would be a good pair of places to focus on. The left shoulder is called the 'tension area' while the right hip is called the 'intention area'. By bringing these two areas into focus, we can visualise a gentle flow of qi away from the tension and encourage greater blood circulation over a larger area of the body. From here, we might then draw focus to the left foot or ankle, to draw blood circulation even further across the body. Throughout this entire process, it is important to maintain a positive, caring, and patient attitude.

Overall, these steps are very powerful for improving and maintaining health. We always start with a caring attitude, then draw tension towards an area of intention. To improve our focus between these two areas, it can be helpful to close the eyes or focus on a breathing rhythm as a regulating pace for circulation. With time, the tension will start to fade, and at this point, we should try to redirect our focus to a second intention area to continue to spread the flow of qi and blood.

It is important to maintain a holistic view, focusing on our entire body and all aspects of life, rather than honing in too much on just one area or aspect. This will maintain a healthy and dynamic flow of qi and blood.

For self-reflection ...

Which areas on the body would you consider to be 'oppositely' or 'distantly' placed from each other? These are areas between which you might be able to visualise an energy flow, especially when you are feeling unwell or are injured in one of these areas.

REAL-LIFE APPLICATIONS

Part 6

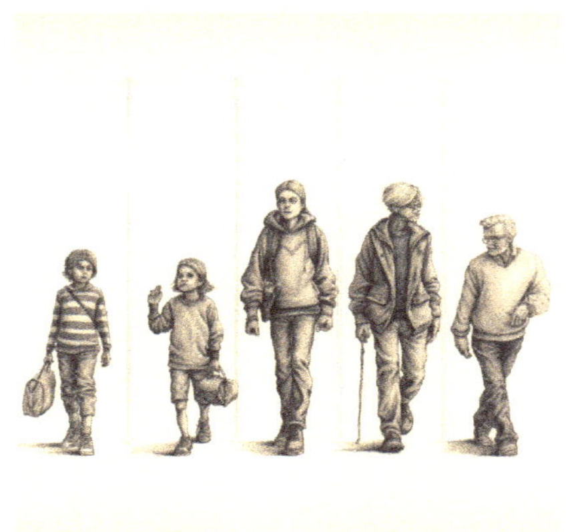

There are many inter-related yet diverse concepts we have covered in this book, and it may feel overwhelming or a little daunting when it comes to applying them to life. It is important to remain patient with oneself, and learn to embrace these new concepts with positivity, understanding, and self-care. In Part 6, we will discuss the concepts and theories in this book in a more realistic context. We have structured this section with different stages of life, ranging from birth to retired life. As you take in these next few chapters, we encourage you to maintain an open mind, and allow yourself to draw connections between the presented ideas and your own life.

BIRTH TO EARLY CHILDHOOD

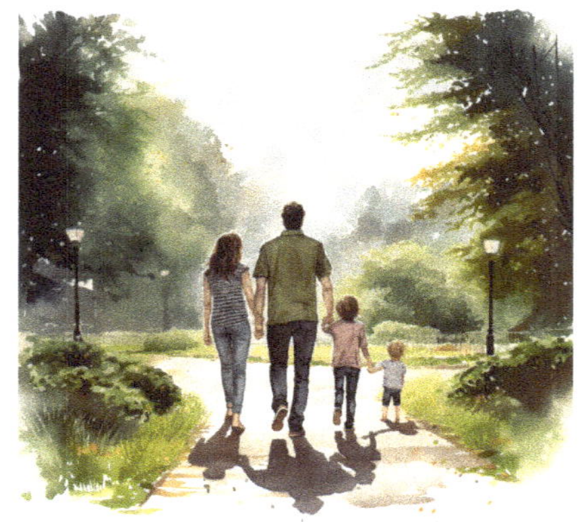

Parents usually bring their very young children to the clinic for concerns surrounding nutrition, eating habits, skin health or sleeping habits. Other concerns include allergies, genetics, digestion, and muscular development. At this age, we often see that we can help both parents and their children equally. As children are not yet strong communicators, their parents are often highly stressed and alert. Parents usually see multiple doctors from various backgrounds of medicine and tend to look to pharmaceutical and contemporary medicine for remedies first. In some cases, parents do not agree completely with caring methods that have been recommended to them in this process, or simply want to take a more natural method of healing, and thus begin engaging with Chinese medicine practices.

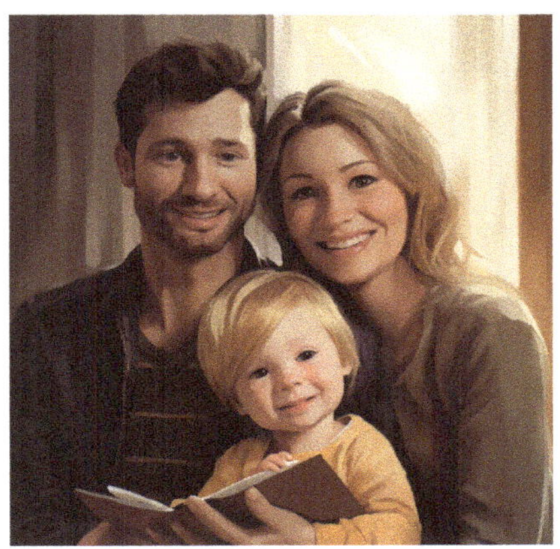

Parents are a major influence on their children all through their children's lives. Even from birth into early childhood, children can sense their parents' stress and alertness, and thus be affected by it. Therefore, with young children, parents may reap the most benefits from applying concepts in Part 2 of this book, *Mind, Connection with the Physical*. When parents can take care of themselves by strengthening their mind-body connection, children will also be able to sense this and benefit from it.

Parents should regularly practice the strategy described in *One Mechanism: Mind, Body, and Breath* (Part 2) to first establish and strengthen their mind-body connection. At moments of stress or conflict, parents should visualise their emotions (as described in *Visibility of Emotions* in Part 2) to bring a greater sense of calm to their mind, continuing to allow their mind-body connection to grow.

Another strategy for coping with stressful situations is practising projecting stress and other negative emotions into the environment, using the mindfulness technique described in *Projecting to the Environment* (Part 2). This technique can be practiced in any space and at any time, and the more it is practiced, the more effective it will become.

PRIMARY SCHOOL

The next stage in a child's life begins when they enter primary school. At this time, children are drawn away from their home environment, which is all they have ever known until this point. This contrast challenges the mind and emotions of a child, and may manifest in the form of head colds that are easily 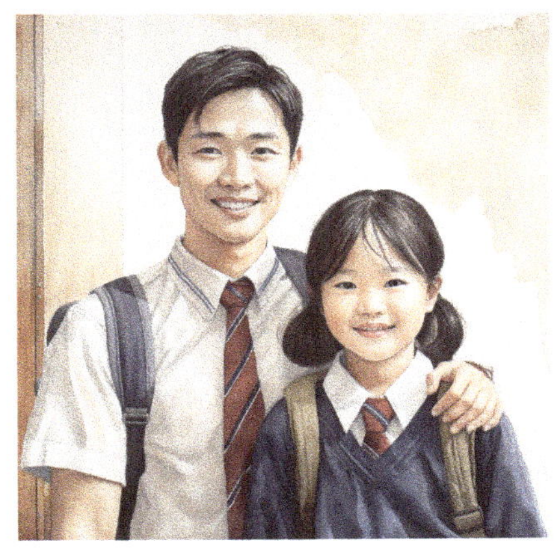 spread. Furthermore, children within this age group may experience mild injuries (such as sprained ankles) as they are introduced to many new distractions in their environment. Children are also prone to behavioural changes as they meet new people and encounter new social situations.

To best support their children and the many new challenges they encounter at this time, parents should apply concepts from *Within Our Environment*, Part 3 of the book. Parents may find that applying concepts in the chapter, *Time and Space* (Part 3), is highly effective. For example, when children are unwell or simply feeling overwhelmed by several new aspects in their environment, parents should focus on providing healing spaces. This is much more important than stressing about the time it may take for their children to recover from illness, or to become acclimated to new situations they are encountering.

During this time, children are gaining more information than materials and energy, which are concepts outlined in the chapter, *The Universe and Flow* (Part 3). Therefore, providing sufficient materials and positive energy for them to navigate all the influx of new information can be helpful. This may simply look like remaining patient with the children and using encouraging words to project positivity. Ideas from the chapter, *Scent in the Environment* (Part 3), may also be beneficial. While heavy use of perfumes or incense may not seem to be best matched to young children, the power of scent as a healing mechanism is still valuable. For example, flower therapy or aromatherapy are both highly accessible ways of creating a healing atmosphere for children. Additionally, these techniques help children find greater harmony with natural scents and their natural environment, encouraging them to see nature as a source of healing in their later lives.

MIDDLE AND HIGH SCHOOL

As children complete their primary years of learning and move through middle and high school, they begin experiencing various new sensations and emotions. For example, their study load increases, their friendships grow stronger, they may play more sports or spend more time with friends. They are likely to experience emotions associated with hormonal changes. Their likes, dislikes and preferences are also strengthening, and their opinions of the world are forming.

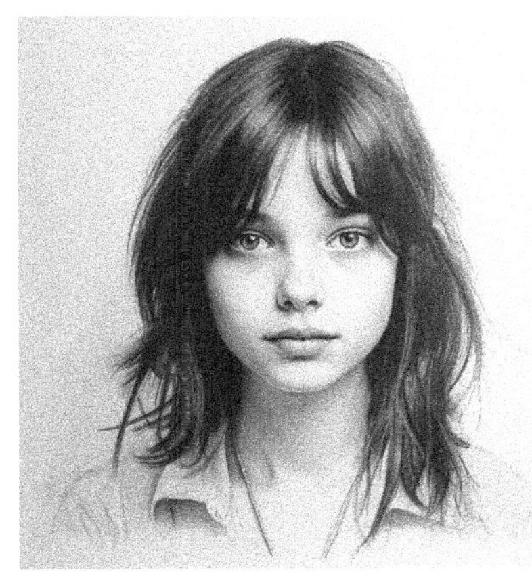

We can see that in various ways, their energy is changing. Therefore, there are many techniques and concepts that may be useful from Part 5 of this book, *Energy*, for both parents and children. If parents or children feel frustrated or stressed, rather than focusing on expressing this pain, they should focus on the sensations of hidden pain that are associated with the emotions. These concepts are described in the chapter, *Types of Pain* (Part 5). Using mindful breathing techniques may help to hone in on this focus on the energy of the emotion rather than the expression of the emotion. This also reduces negative energy that may be spread to others.

Concepts in the chapter, *Literature and Energy* (Part 5), may also be applicable to this age group. Using positive communication methods and varying words and sentence structures will promote a healthier variety of energy levels that are projected during conversations. Again, this will encourage more flowing, positive energy and less rigid, negative energy in social settings.

Especially with their study workload increasing, teenagers may find that they are spending more time sitting down. As described in the chapter, *Yin and Yang in Body Positions* (Part 5), this can become harmful as yin and yang energies become stagnant and do not flow well in this position. Therefore, en-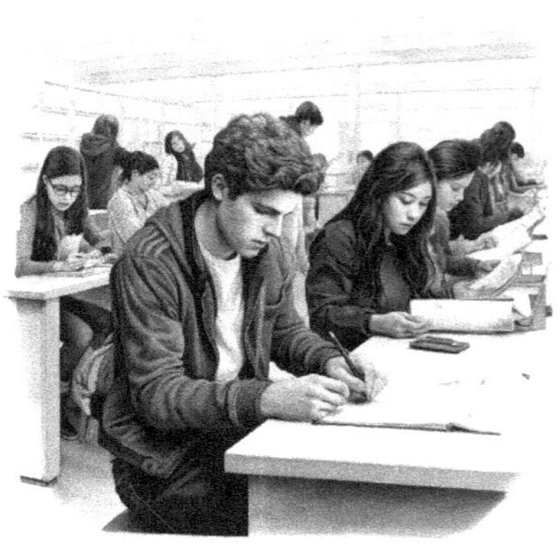couraging kids to remain active and find a healthy balance between study, physical activity, and leisure activities is very important and valuable.

UNIVERSITY AND START OF WORK

Following on from high school, young adults often choose to begin studies at the university-level or start to work. Both pathways signify a grand first step towards influencing society. With this first step, stress can emerge from the increase of responsibilities, change of lifestyle, and pressure of making career-defining decisions.

Parents are also less able to support young adults. At this time, young adults are often moving out of their parents' home or becoming more independent. Parents of young adults studying at the university-level are also usually no longer able to support their children with their academic learning, as the difficulty of study begins to advance enormously.

As a result of all these changing factors, young adults may experience changes to their sleeping habits, diet, or exercise, and are much more prone to experiencing stress, anxiety, lethargy, depression, and other general symptoms of poorer mental health. Being new to so many new responsibilities can make it difficult for young adults to reflect on themselves and find help to improve their situation.

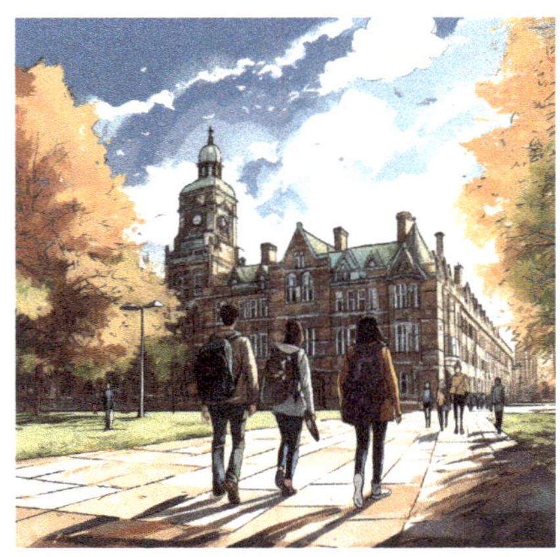

We can draw many beneficial connections between the experiences of this age group and Part 1 of this book, which is about the *Structure of the Body*. For example, in the chapter, *Structure and Our Control* (Part 1), young adults can apply the discussed concepts to better comprehend how their level of control over their wellbeing relates to different areas of the body. Using theory from the chapter, *Three Vertical Planes* (Part 1), young adults can also learn more about how to maintain balance between their scientific, logical self and their more mindful, intuitive self, in order to keep grounded and healthy overall. The ideas in the chapter, *Posture and Body Language* (Part 1), will help young adults to understand their most dominant elements more deeply and how to use physical movement and body posture to re-instate balance between the elements. Furthermore, young adults should focus on their future health by applying techniques from the chapter, *Interaction Between the Face and Abdomen* (Part 1). Due to the rapidly changing lifestyles of young adults, thinking forward about health will help to prevent illness or injury in future, and may improve mental health more sustainably.

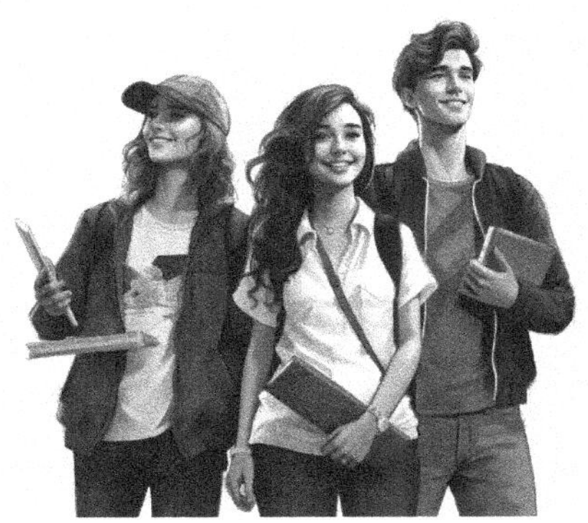

At this age, young adults can understand themselves on a deeper and more complex level than at younger ages. They are able to analyse their body structure and elemental composition. These concepts are quite intricate, but understanding and being able to reflect on them can be valuable for their health.

POST-GRADUATION AND IMMERSION IN THE WORK FORCE

Post graduation, or following on from entrance into the workforce, adults are further immersed into work and delve into their careers and adult life. Some find this time of life to be much different from their expectations, especially regarding their career expectations. This induces stress, which relates to new environments, new relationships, the possibility of starting or planning for a family, and simply being quite busy with new work. Energy levels can oscillate according to the situation.

Adults at this time want to learn, adapt, and establish themselves as accomplished individuals, but there is a mental barrier of uncertainty that can make this difficult. This may be the uncertainty of the future, of relationships, or of career changes, for example. Having uncertainty is natural, and we should be accepting of this and embrace it in order to continue healing sustainably. Therefore, we should apply concepts from Part 4 of this book, *Sustainable Healing*.

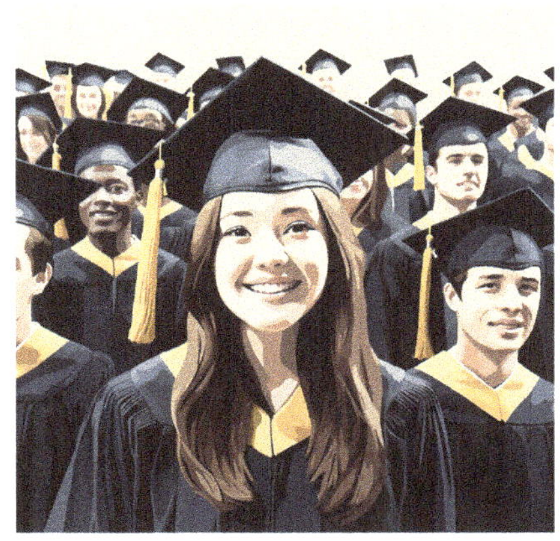

In the chapter, *Sustainability* (Part 4), we discussed the importance of not using full force in the direction of our intention, and holding some reserved effort within us. This further reinforces that we should be accepting of and embrace our uncertainty, as this can act as a reserved force that keeps us balanced and healthy. Additionally, we should learn and understand more about the elements and how we relate to them. In this way, the chapters, *Balance of Elements* and *Two Cycles of Five Elements* (Part 4), may be most useful. The first of these two chapters discusses the meaning of balance and the second describes how we can work to regulate balance between the elements.

The chapter, *Levels of Healing* (Part 4), will also be helpful by providing a strategy for seeing the world in the most logical way, without getting lost in our inner stress and worry. Additionally, the chapter, *Aspects Influencing General Health* (Part 4), will also provide useful guidance regarding maintaining general health and wellbeing.

MAJOR ADULT LIFE

Our major adult life begins when we have achieved a greater level of stability in life. During the major adult life period, an individual may have a growing family, senior parents, or young children. They may also be at the mid-point of their career, with lots of responsibilities and less time to do activities other than work.

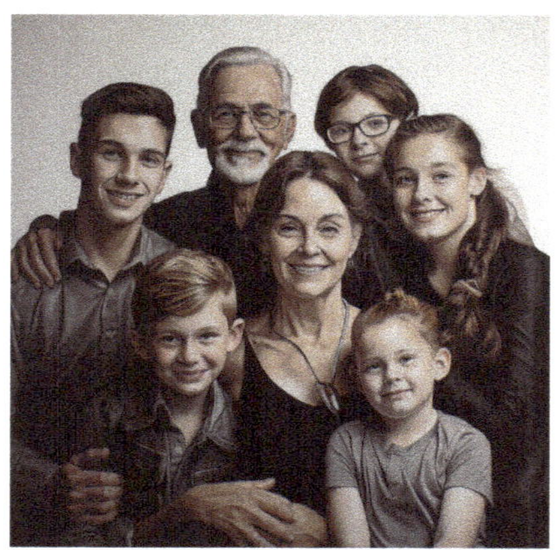

At this stage of life, it is much more difficult to assign a most useful part of this book in terms of guiding concepts and theories. Rather, all the parts of this book are relevant to this period.

For example, understanding one's constitution and dominant elements can greatly inform our decisions surrounding health and wellbeing. Hence, the chapters, *Balance of Elements* (Part 4) and *Two Cycles of Five Elements* (Part 4), may be useful. It is also important to note that our constitution and dominant elements may vary between different stages of life. Therefore, this is an understanding upon which we should continue reflecting throughout life.

Sometimes during this period, we may also feel quite rigid or inflexible due to strict structures and timeframes in our day-to-day lives, especially as we are at a point when many people depend on us. This can affect our ability to adapt well or make good decisions. In this case, we should practice more mindfulness and breathing techniques, which are discussed in the chapter, *One Mechanism: Mind, Body, and Breath* (Part 2).

We can also work with our flow of energy and qi on which the chapter, *Openness, Closedness, and Transition* (Part 5), provides significant guidance.

RETIRED LIFE

The final main stage of life is that of retirement. By this stage, we have already completed the bulk of our work, and usually find the need to slow down and take more time for ourselves. We can see some balance across our life from youth to old age. For example, when we are young, we are much more energetic and full of life, yet we are less knowledgeable. When we reach old age, we tend to be more physically limited, while our minds are still very active, and full of wisdom.

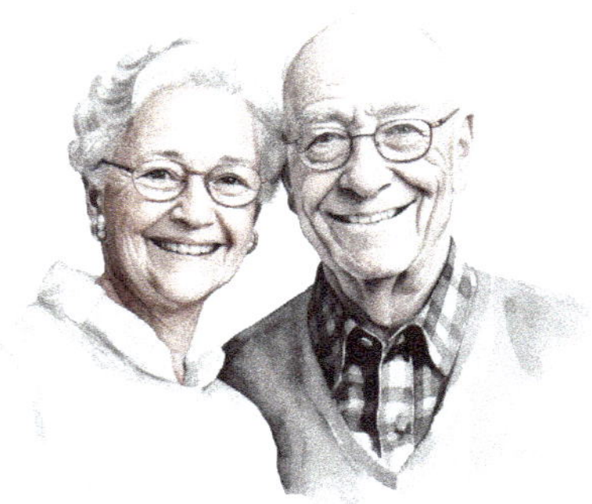

Spirituality and the mind are at its peak at this time. Therefore, health issues and challenges that arise earlier in life now have the opportunity to heal themselves through the power of the mind. The most important thing we can do to help this process, is to embrace our spirituality and be welcoming towards healing.

It is at this stage that we are also able to embrace passion at the highest level. Though this stage is much later in life, it is the time at which we can be open to greater passion and emotion. Through techniques that develop mind-body connection, we can shift this passion into wellbeing, health, and happiness.

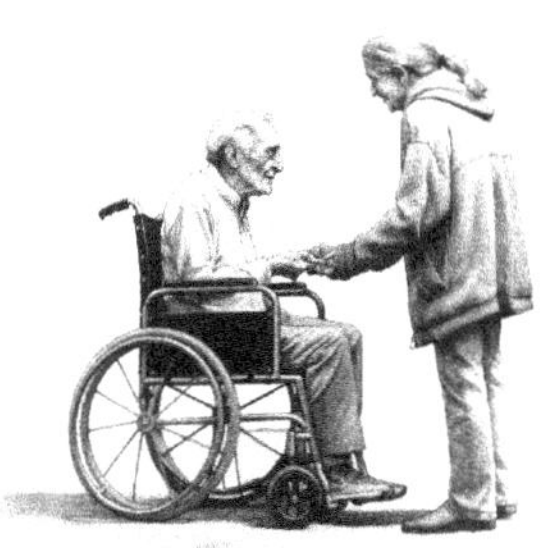

At the very end of the retirement age, we approach the end of life. This may involve moving into nursing homes or hospice care, and we may experience terminal diseases or major debilitation. At this point, all the concepts in this book are applicable and the power of healing holistically is prominent. We should revisit key concepts that span across this book as they are all beneficial during this time, such as the structure of the body, mind-body partnership, energy, and the environment.

It should be noted that it is not necessary to understand every concept in every chapter of this book. This book provides guidance and knowledge, but truthfully, much of this is already within you, and the book serves only as a reminder of the power already within you to improve your health, happiness, and wellbeing. 'I Know You Know' is a book of connection, and sees healing as an art and beauty. Eventually, everything we experience has a way of interacting with other aspects of life, and often has a way of healing itself through kindness and appreciation.

Dr Haisong Wang

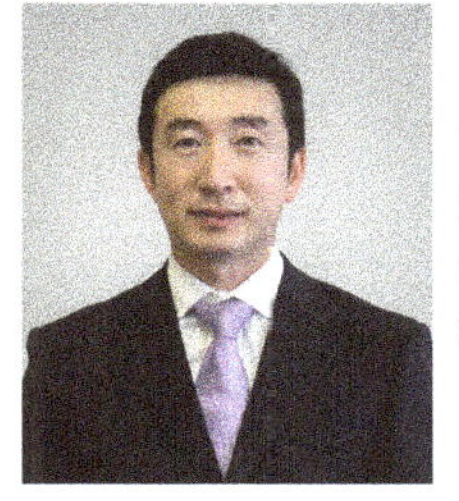

Dr Haisong Wang is a Chinese medicine and tai chi practitioner, and has been practising at his family-owned clinic, Capital Health Centre of Traditional Chinese Medicine, in Canberra, Australia, since 2000.

Prior to this, Dr Haisong worked in the emergency department of a hospital in China. He also taught Technical and Further Education (TAFE) courses in Chinese medicine at the Canberra Institute of Technology (CIT) from 1999 to 2009.

Now, while practicing at his clinic, Dr Haisong is involved in various projects with his staff members, with the focus of promoting health and wellbeing within the Canberra community and beyond. Dr Haisong's projects often stem from shared interests and motivations with his clients and develop into meaningful collaborations. He has developed projects and talk-groups with various members of the community, and from various backgrounds of health and other expertise.

He has a Bachelor's degree in Chinese Medicine and a Master's degree in Prescription Science in Chinese Herbal Medicine from Liaoning University of Traditional Chinese Medicine.

Pryor Hollis

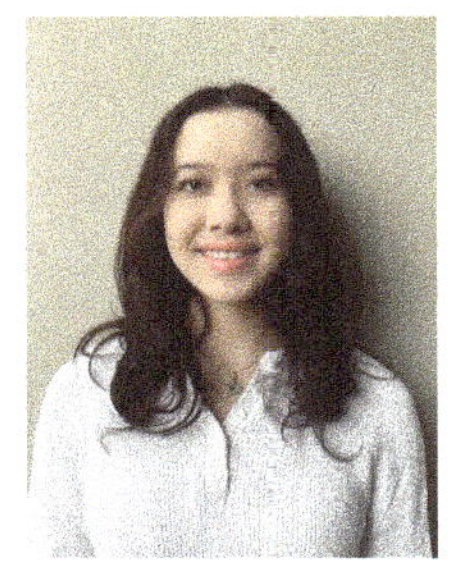

Pryor Hollis is studying full-time at the Australian National University (ANU), working towards a Bachelor of Science degree. She primarily studies physics, mathematics, and French.

Pryor is passionate about supporting her worldwide community. In 2022, she planned and coordinated fundraising and awareness-raising events and several college-level workshops for, and in collaboration with, organisations against human trafficking, Blue Dragon Children's Foundation and The Human, Earth Project. The events included a film-screening and QnA session open to the Canberra community, and brought to light the horrors and immense challenges that human trafficking in Vietnam represents.

She is also a passionate advocate for women in STEM and values the arts, particularly dance and music.

Pryor works part-time as a personal assistant and administrative staff member at the Capital Health Centre of Traditional Chinese Medicine in Canberra. Her broad interests and global perspective bring diversity to the clinic, through various projects she works on with other staff members surrounding health and wellbeing in the community.

www.ingramcontent.com/pod-product-compliance
Lightning Source LLC
Chambersburg PA
CBHW050027040726